Health Crisis
2000

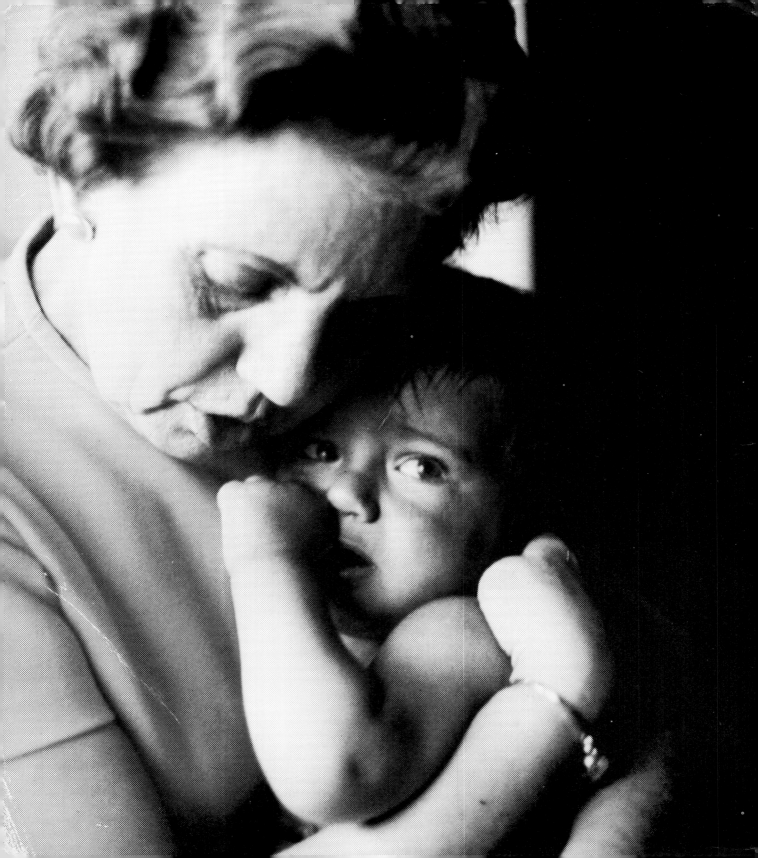

Health Crisis 2000

Peter O'Neill

Foreword by the Rt. Hon. Dr. David Owen MP

Published for the
World Health Organization Regional Office for Europe
Copenhagen

William Heinemann Medical Books Ltd and
William Heinemann Ltd · London

Acknowledgements

HEALTH CRISIS 2000 would not have seen the light of day without the encouragement of Dr Leo A. Kaprio, WHO Regional Director for Europe, and the sound advice of WHO's European Programme Director Dr Jo Asvall. Martin Jones, WHO Publications Officer, who worked closely on the book with me, gave unstintingly of his time and ideas, as did all his staff. My wife, Uma Ram Nath, was no less willing with her time and editorial expertise. The other officers and consultants at WHO in Copenhagen, whose work I drew on heavily, were mines of information and help, and their commitment to a policy of Health for All by the Year 2000 was a constant reminder of the vital issues at stake. Finally, my thanks to all those WHO staff who, at every hour of the day and night, were ready to help unscramble the havoc that I wrought on the text processing system, and so helped produce the final manuscript.

Peter O'Neill   1983

About the author

Peter O'Neill, BA (Joint Hons), M.Phil., 37, is an English freelance journalist in London. The feature agency he runs with his Indian wife, THIRD WORLD: EEC, concentrates on international issues and the work of the United Nations and its specialist agencies. His interest in WHO's work first began when he was a Reuter correspondent in India during the historic WHO smallpox eradication programme. Their broadcasting and writing include regular contributions on health issues affecting the developed and developing world.

The views expressed in this book are those of the author, and do not necessarily represent the decisions or the stated policy of the World Health Organization.

First published in a limited edition by
the World Health Organization, 1982

This edition first published 1983
© The World Health Organization 1983
ISBN 0-433-24011-3 (cased)
ISBN 0-433-24010-5 (paper)

Printed in Great Britain by the Alden Press, Oxford

Contents

Foreword

The future of the industrial nations' welfare states is plagued by doubts. The outward signs are conflict over cash allocations, private versus public medicine and political ideology. But all this hides a more dangerous and fundamental problem. The successes of the welfare state have also produced the attitudes of the jailer, affecting individuals and the community. "Health" has become institutionalized, a problem to "cure", rather than a state of mind and body to promote.

The World Health Organization, which commissioned this book and whose greatest achievements have been in the field of public medicine, is right in warning every industrialized nation that there will be a *Health Crisis* unless they embark on a programme of radical change. This must be a cross-party political issue and across the different health related disciplines too. We can no more entrust it exclusively to the politicians than we can to the medical profession to offer a "cure" for this illness. True health extends far beyond the powers of politicians or of those who work in the health field. Every one of us must take and demand preventive action to halt, for example, the epidemic of road traffic accidents which slaughters our children, or industrial diseases which emerge too late because of inadequate research. The law can help. But only through public opinion and fresh attitudes can industrial society heal itself of the new social diseases – illness from tobacco, alcohol and narcotics or the psychological scarring and callousness of a culture which turns away from its elderly. The handicapped and the mentally ill will be all too frequently social lepers in the 21st century on present trends.

Medical progress has been immense. But the great strides in public health emerged from social movements leading to good sanitary engineering, free education and the elimination of much poverty and poor housing. Today, unemployment affects tens of millions and poverty and illness are increasing. A new social movement is needed to question the way scientific ingenuity, spurred on by unthinking consumer demand and profit, has corrupted our political, economic, industrial and social lifestyles. This book, written to be accessible to all, analyses the crux of the crisis and outlines WHO's strategic response. Not least, it argues for more political "health power" for women who carry the burden of family and self-care. The health of a nation touches every nerve and muscle in society, so reform must be born out of public debate and participation. This book will serve as a vital catalyst in that process.

The Rt. Hon. Dr. David Owen MP

Preface

This book is based on the WHO European Regional Strategy for Attaining Health for All by the Year 2000. When the Strategy was formally adopted by the 33 Member States of the European Region it was felt that a dramatic book about the issues involved would enable a larger audience to participate in the dialogue as to what the real issues are. I am happy to note that the author has succeeded in writing such a book by enlarging the scope of the document to include illustrations, facts and figures, and concrete examples.

The book is, of course, no longer the Regional Strategy document as approved by the Member States; it is a text about it. The Strategy itself, however, has evolved from discussions among the Regional Office staff, health experts, and the European governments. It will continue to evolve as its targets are reached one by one and as conditions change. An essential feature of the Strategy and its development is public participation, and therein lies the strength of this book. I am confident that it will stimulate the public debate and political decisions which are essential if we are to attain our goal of health for all.

Leo A. Kaprio
Regional Director, WHO

Introduction

As Europe enters the last two decades of the 20th century, the WHO Regional Office for Europe has no option but to warn that there could be a health crisis by the year 2000 unless radical steps are taken by the public, the professions, industry, and the governments of the Region. This is no idle warning. A careful analysis of trends in health and disease, made over the past three years by representatives of the medical profession and the health ministries of the Region's 33 Member States, has produced ominous signs that our health policies since the Second World War have set us on a dangerous course.

The glittering attraction of high technology and the public's demand for "miracle cures" have meant that we have almost abandoned the principle of self-care in a "caring community". We have inflicted wounds on ourselves, in the belief that science, doctors and hospitals would find a cure, instead of preventing the very causes of illness in the first place. Of course we cannot do without the medical care facilities that actually save life, but let us be clear that they do not add to our "health" — they stop us dying. Hospitals can only "cure" probably between 10% and 20% of disease. Instead of promoting health and preventing disease, we have invested the bulk of our health budgets in "disease palaces" which have really only cured our acute illnesses. Moreover, some countries have not only built hospitals that are too expensive for the return they give in terms of health; they have also built too many.

Malaria, smallpox, typhoid, cholera — some of the great plagues of mankind — hold no mystery for modern medicine, but cancer, heart disease, the self-destructive urge of the smoker and the drinker, the effects on mind and body of unemployment — these are some of the "new diseases". Why do we allow the "road accident epidemic", which plunders lives and drains our financial resources? It diverts medical resources that should be spent on the chronic diseases of old age and in rehabilitating our handicapped and mentally ill; its continuation is sheer social and economic madness.

We must be grateful for the amazing advances that medical science has made in the last 100 years, but the way governments have neglected planning and invested badly, and the way the individual and the community have ignored health has meant that the most important research, that on promoting health and preventing illness, has been left largely undone. If we are to avoid the crisis, and it will certainly come if we stand idle, then we must begin now to make radical changes in the way health is won and medical care provided.

We must honestly assess whether we are tricking ourselves by continuing the development of enormously expensive technology to deal with, say, heart disease, when good primary health and medical care, by and for the individual and the community, could reduce the risk of most heart afflictions. The great medical research challenges of the next 20 years must be to find out why we have our "modern diseases", and how much they are due to the way we live and the environment we are creating around us. Only the foolish would say we do not need science, technology and research. We do need them — but in the right place, and at the right time. High technology should be part of an efficient referral system. Research should help us understand how we can keep healthy and prevent illness, not just cure it.

These new diseases do not have miracle cures, but we can do a great deal to tackle their causes. While we must avoid prescribing a common plan of attack, there are certain basic steps which every country in the Region can take, and there is much they can do together. If we are to attain health for all by the year 2000 we must seek to implement a new strategy, one that has three inseparable themes running through it:

— health as a way of life

— the prevention of ill health

— community care for all.

This book is about the implications of such a strategy that has been drawn up for WHO's European Region. The Strategy document itself (EUR/RC30/8 Rev.2) is a short summary version of research results and discussions that have taken place over the last three years. It contains a framework for action, whereas this book spells out more fully for debate the background to our present problems and those steps which must be taken to avoid a crisis.

The three strands of the Strategy in fact represent a political credo, which emphasizes the value of the individual in a caring family and community framework. The implication is that health is the responsibility of the whole state and all its citizens.

First, by reappraising our lifestyles, we can become conscious of our health and spread the idea of health as a way of life. Illness is often caused by neglecting those factors in our daily lives over which we could have complete control *if we wished to exercise it*. We must also try to bring about a greater health awareness — of the ill effects of smoking, excessive consumption of alcohol and indeed the excessive consumption of medicines themselves. The producing industries must take their share of the responsibility too, or bow to legislation by public demand.

The second stage is to prevent disease or reduce risk. That means immunizing all our children, but it also means making childbearing a safer and more natural time for mother and child alike. It means a real plan to cut road accidents, particularly among adolescents, and accidents in the home where women, children and the elderly take the brunt. This can work only if the people at risk actually have a say in deciding how we develop this part of community care. We must all rediscover and stimulate primary health care, giving it a new role, so that it is capable of dealing with these emerging health concerns in a way which makes for a new partnership between the people and the health care providers.

This is not offered as a politician's catch-phrase to justify cuts in health expenditure. A participating and caring community should allow much more effective use of resources. This brings us to that third strand of the Strategy: ensuring that people have access to health care at whatever level they need it. At the moment, the system is overburdened at the top, and a minor illness that should be tackled effectively at the first sign, too often becomes a major problem in a hospital where, frankly, it is really rather late. Resources must be channelled towards preventing illness in the first place and to manage, rather than try to cure, some of the new diseases. This can be achieved by creating a community-oriented health system where a health team — which means more than just the traditional family doctor — is responsive and responsible to the local community, serves its needs, and actively promotes good health.

The growth of active local, regional and national commissions or councils of health system users will also determine community care. That means the involvement of every sector of society — including housing officials and builders, industrialists and food producers, young people, the elderly and the disabled. This is because each in its own way actually influences the kind of health that society has. We have tended to think of health as simply the reverse of illness, for which a doctor or perhaps a hospital means cure — or death. No! Health also means the industrialist ensuring he does not pollute the rivers that provide our drinking-water; it means everyone eliminating poverty — the worst cause of ill health — and governments acting to cut unemployment. Too few people realize that unemployment actually severely increases illness and death.

It would seem wise that women should acquire an important role in these commissions. They are the biggest users of the health system because of their key role in developing family life, and they usually have to pick up the pieces of the shattered health of their family members.

This political role will also enable them to get society as a whole to recognize the fact that they carry the major burden in society.

This political framework of participation and decision-making must be eased into acceptability among both the medical and the political professions. It is perhaps no fault of doctors that they have come to acquire — and indeed the public has helped impose it on them — a status that has alienated them from the very people they most wish to serve. However, they have to some extent been willing to fall in line with what has been almost a social fetish for the development of specializations. The consequent demand for unnecessarily sophisticated and ever more costly equipment and research often turns the patient into an assortment of disconnected nuts and bolts, when the first essential is to view him as a whole personality interacting with a highly complex social and working environment.

We therefore need to harness the skills of the medical professional to bring about a change in training based, for example, on the community rather than the hospital. This will mean sharing understanding of medical affairs with nurses, social workers, health visitors, midwives and the public. It offers a great challenge to society, and the medical profession can be the catalyst.

We now need a whole new approach to what constitutes health and government. Health ministries must not be looked on as cure operations. Other ministries, such as those concerned with transport, housing, industry and trade, can become potent weapons for a healthy society if they only realize that what they do has a direct bearing on people's health. The unemployed man may be depressed, but a pill is almost a dishonest way to tackle his problem — he needs a job.

Any caring community must also ensure a high quality of life for those most at risk. These people may be handicapped, mentally or physically; or they may be wise but old in years and afflicted with the diseases of old age. For a Region with so large and growing a population of elderly people as Europe, the disease of isolation and social rejection has become a curse and threat to a nation's health. So have the inexorably damaging effects of long-term unemployment among the fit, and particularly the young. These are social diseases that have a frightening impact on our lives — and they do not respond to antibiotics.

Here is something that the industrialized North can learn from the traditional values of the countries of the South, both in Europe and throughout the world. The values of the extended family, where age brings respect and care not isolation and rejection, must be rediscovered. The challenge of Health for All by the Year 2000 must never be allowed to be prostituted into the crude battle-cry of "heart transplants for all". This is a global challenge and part of that fundamental re-organization of human relationships in the world through the search for a New International Economic Order, whereby all look forward to the future together, not in opposition to each other.

This is a time for decisions, because time is short. Many of these problems cannot be solved by one country alone and we need to work out a health policy for Europe. We need targets and dates to reduce alcoholism and smoking. That means we need public support and political decisions. We may find that we shall need a kind of European "manifesto for health" which cuts across party boundaries and political differences among heads of state, but which all can back in the spotlight of the political arena.

This book analyses the first stage of the work which the WHO European Region has drawn up for itself. It is part of a Global Strategy for Health for All, which gathered speed at the Conference on Primary Health Care held in Alma-Ata in September 1978. Since then the Regional Office has been working with the Member States to draw up a battle plan; this book is about that plan and the Strategy for success. However, the day has gone when the health profession and the legislators could do the job alone − this Strategy can work only if the public implement it. The Regional Office therefore commissioned this book to interpret for a wider audience the official document on the Regional Strategy for Attaining Health for All by the Year 2000. Inspired by documentation from the Region's Member States and the Regional Committee for Europe, this book provides ample detail and challenge to draw ministers, parliamentarians, industrialists and the media into the debate. If, through the media and from political platforms, the public too become involved, then I believe we shall soon see the goal of Health for All becoming one of the great issues for public debate and action in this century.

Peter O'Neill
London, 1983

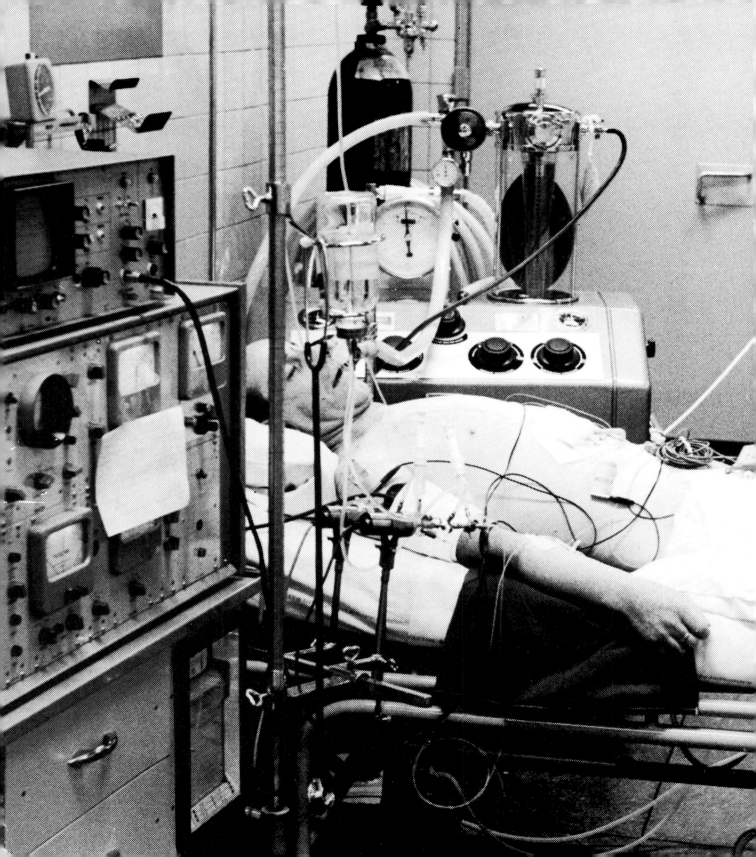

1.

The origins of the impending crisis

THE DRAMA OF MEDICAL PROGRESS

In the years since the Second World War the vast increase in resources devoted to health care have enabled the richer countries of the European Region[a] to take advantage of the progress in biomedical research. This has produced a whole new range of effective drugs and high-technology medical equipment. The benefits derived by particular groups of patients from these advances have been immense. There has been an enormous increase in the standard of physical care and comfort provided for the acutely sick and, though to a much lesser extent, for the disabled. Yet only 30 years ago tuberculosis was a major cause of death, the periodic ravages of poliomyelitis left behind them a trail of permanently disabled young people, and even measles killed hundreds of children every year. The virtual conquest of the major killing infectious diseases in the high-income countries of the Region has been a great achievement. In the poorer countries of the Region there has also been a major improvement in health standards — fewer mothers die in childbirth and more children survive to maturity. The expectation of life at birth in some countries has increased by ten or more years.

The growing domination of medicine by the big, technologically sophisticated hospitals is, however, a recent phenomenon, particularly in the treatment of the acutely sick. Progress in anaesthetics and asepsis, in new surgical procedures and drugs has made possible the treatment of the very sick, who in the past could look forward only to death or a miserable existence. However, the successes of modern medicine are familiar to most Europeans. Everyone knows that his living conditions are healthier and that he can expect to live much longer than his grandparents. There has, however, been a bias towards the development of hospitals rather than care in the community, and towards curative rather than preventive medicine. The public, encouraged by doctors and led by politicians, has demanded hospitals. Their presence in every city was taken to be a symbol of "modern civilization". In fact they have often destroyed the personal relationship between doctor and patient and made a crucial contribution to the loss of the real meaning of health as something to be enjoyed rather than merely the absence of illness.

---

[a] As at 31 December 1980 the European Region of the World Health Organization had 33 active Member States, namely: Albania, Algeria, Austria, Belgium, Bulgaria, Czechoslovakia, Denmark, Finland, France, German Democratic Republic, Federal Republic of Germany, Greece, Hungary, Iceland, Ireland, Italy, Luxembourg, Malta, Monaco, Morocco, Netherlands, Norway, Poland, Portugal, Romania, San Marino, Spain, Sweden, Switzerland, Turkey, USSR, United Kingdom and Yugoslavia.

This analysis of the situation is not meant to apportion blame to any particular group in society. We have all been to blame for not standing back to see where we were going. Some members of the medical profession may feel that the responsibility has been mainly theirs. That would not be true because in fact both the public and the health professions are trapped within the same straitjacket of the high-technology, hospital-based society. It is this which prevents them from working together and focusing on the search for community health.

In this and the next two chapters medical developments and other social change, like all "progress" are seen to have their price. Medical progress has not been an unqualified success: benefits have also brought problems. The costs of high technology have been high and often inappropriate. Government departments, often under public pressure, have taken a narrow view and subordinated the overall interest to their own sectional interests, which has led to poor planning and unbalanced investment. The "new diseases" of modern society are briefly described, and the careless social attitudes that have emerged are outlined. A discussion on the loss of caring in the community concludes this bleak survey of self-created problems that are leading us into a health crisis. The book then continues with a strategy for dealing with them to achieve the completely feasible goal of health for all by the year 2000.

THE COSTS OF TECHNOLOGY

High technology in the medical field today falls within three broad categories. These are: laboratory support, radiology (from the humble X-ray for a fracture to the nuclear medicine services for tracking isotopes through the blood system) and the various life support and monitoring systems for the cardiac surgery patient, the crash victim, or the premature baby. There has been a steep rise in the cost of providing and running these services over the last 20 years. Research and industrial development have led to rapid progress and increased sophistication in the technology, but also to much higher costs and to increased sales pressure to buy the latest product. Public opinion, reflected in the media, must share the blame for the voracious demand for such equipment, and the medical profession has been happy to go along.

The inflation of the system has continued as health authorities have created new medical units, sometimes mainly in response to political pressure and without any prior close investigation of the need for them. These units have not always been suitably staffed, equipped or used, and the service has been of low quality. The result has often been an almost complete waste of money and, more important, a failure to supply the better health service that was supposed to be the prime motive.

Table 1. Cost of health care (in millions of guilders) in the Netherlands, 1973–1977

	Year				
	1973[a]	1974	1975	1976	1977[a]
Inpatient health care	6 663 (55)	8 060	9 749	11 222	12 519 (58)
Specialist assistance[b]	970 (8)	1 110	1 261	1 346	1 484 (7)
Medicaments and prosthetics	1 500 (12)	1 640	1 855	2 025	2 174 (10)
Outpatient health care	1 961 (16)	2 293	2 668	3 076	3 486 (16)
Community preventive care	323 (3)	372	431	530	581 (3)
Health care in policy-making, administration and management	778 (6)	912	1 028	1 149	1 273 (6)
Total	12 195	14 387	16 992	19 348	21 517

[a] Figures in parentheses indicate percentage of total health costs.

[b] Gross fees for registered free specialists.

Source: Ministry of Health and Environmental Protection (*1*).

Paying at the wrong end of the system. An explosive growth in health care costs is typical of Europe today. In the Netherlands, for example, costs have almost doubled in five years. More than half of these vast sums go to expensive hospitals; only 3% is spent on preventive work in the community.

Table 2. Laboratory testing in general hospitals in the Netherlands, 1973–1977

	Year				
	1973	1974	1975	1976	1977
Laboratory tests per 100 patients	7 323	8 038	9 146	9 952	10 670
Laboratory tests per 100 outpatient visits	597.6	644	729	723.2	767.9

Source: Ministry of Health and Environmental Protection (*1*).

Are all those tests really necessary? Laboratory testing in hospitals is just one area where high-cost technology is over-used. If you go to hospital today the chances are that you will have more than 100 tests during your stay. Even for outpatients the figure has risen in five years from six tests per visit to an average of nearly eight.

4

If we take the use of medical equipment in hospitals as an example, we can see some of the unhappy results. Thirty years ago there were fewer medical instruments, and a community hospital could manage with one or two technically trained people to look after relatively simple items such as X-ray machines. However, the vast increase in inventions and innovations produced new equipment that required more maintenance and more technical expertise. This advancing technology encouraged new medical developments and these, in turn, created a demand for further instruments. The result has been a complex range of sophisticated equipment depending on a technology in which few people have had any training.

At present more than 500 types of test are routinely carried out in approximately 65 000 health care laboratories in the Region and there are a further 500 types for more special health problems. New techniques and costly apparatus have been, and continue to be, introduced, often without proper assessment of their relative benefits (2).

INAPPROPRIATE TECHNOLOGY

Technology in medical care not only often lacks the right staff to use or maintain it but also, because it is developed for use in hospitals, is almost always for the specialist and not for the general practitioner. There is, therefore, no easy access to it by the public. However, this high-technology approach, whether relating to equipment or to drugs, has had even more serious consequences. The aim has been to tackle the health problems that have arrived in the waiting-rooms of doctors and, of course, the hospitals. The aim has certainly not been to prevent health problems from arising in the first place, let alone to seek out those who are at greatest risk of suffering from these problems. Thus, the emphasis has been on cure or remedial treatment, all too often in a hospital, rather than on promoting health and preventing illness. This is confirmed by national expenditures on curative medicine, which are usually many times those on preventive medicine (3). People have come to believe that it is health professionals using technology who can look after them; they do not try to discover how to look after themselves when there is still the time and opportunity to do so. We have ended up with too much high technology, which costs too much and usually is in the wrong place so that, even for those who do obtain access to it, it is often too late.

Unchecked technological development actually results in an increase in certain problems, including hospital infections, accidents due to the excessive use of dangerous diagnostic and therapeutic methods, and adverse effects from drugs. It increases the professional monopoly of health knowledge and reduces self-reliance. The sales promotion practices of some manufacturers also encourage excessive use of tests, drugs, and other forms of medical intervention.

Unfortunately advances in medicine and the provision of new health services rarely produce a demand for greater community care. They merely create a demand for more of the same. The trouble is that more money to "cure" disease and ill health is less effective than money spent to prevent it in the first instance. Therefore, in the long run, you spend more money and get less health. Increased knowledge has often led to too much specialization in medicine and to the largely uncontrolled proliferation and fragmentation of the health services. This, in turn, has led many countries to develop what amounts to *disintegrated* systems of health care dominated entirely by specialists. There is a serious lack of coordination among health services, with a notable absence of links between primary and specialist, outpatient and inpatient care. Coverage of people's health needs has suffered and resources and manpower have been wasted. Worse, the public's expectations have constantly grown, influenced often by considerations far removed from those of good health care (*4*).

Underprivileged, underserved and unprotected minorities. Migrant workers, like one-parent families and the unemployed, tend to get inadequate health care.

THE NARROW VIEWS OF GOVERNMENT DEPARTMENTS

By allowing themselves to be led by the enormous pressures to find "miracle cures" governments, in the form of politicians and the civil servants who staff the various ministries, have come to assume that the main job of the ministry of health is to make sick people get better. It is the ministry of labour or social affairs that is usually responsible for social security. This has led to a failure to recognize the extent to which health depends upon policies in other fields: the economy, agriculture, transport, education, and the environment at home and in the workplace. The view of each ministry has been so restricted that government and ministries have too often ignored the fact that almost every aspect of government policy contains a critical health element.

POOR PLANNING

There has been a lack of planning and coordination between ministries not only because of the obvious conflicts of interests and goals, but also because it was felt that only the ministry of health should respond to health problems, and then only as they arise. This has meant that health systems have been too much characterized by a hit-and-miss approach. Only in a minority of countries have the health services evolved as a planned system. Even in some of the most economically advanced countries of the Region there is no consistent distribution of referral facilities by geographical area according to the needs of the population. There are no clear health policies, no effective structure for health planning, and no adequate system for assessing the real value of new development plans or how they are put into effect.

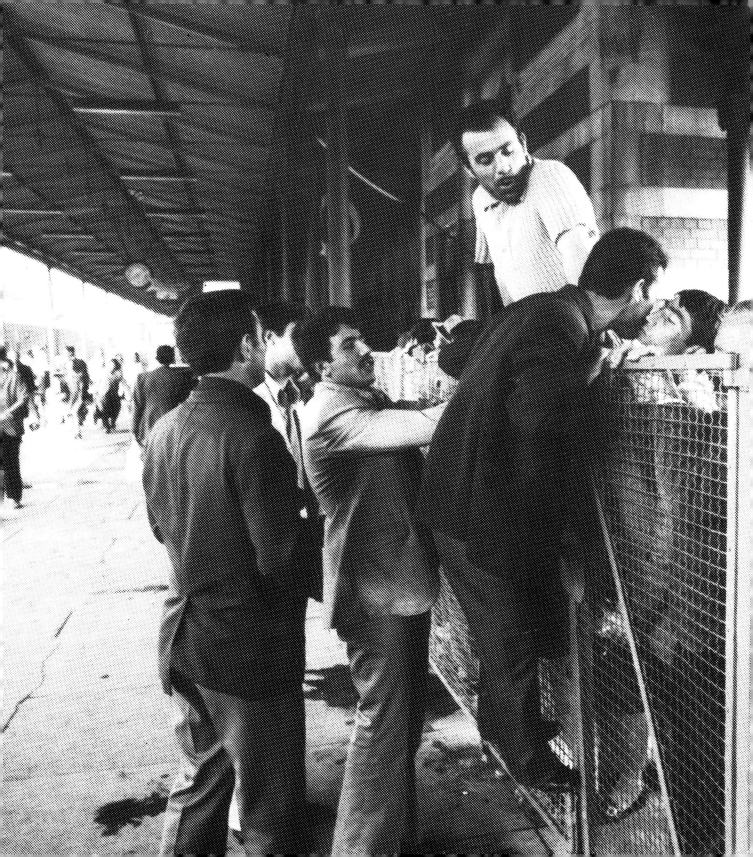

Social security systems have often developed simply as a mechanism for payment under contracts made with a host of separate, fragmented providers: individual professionals, and hospitals under various patterns of ownership. Moreover, some systems of health and social security financing are so structured that they respond only to demands: they pay only when a doctor treats a patient. They do not pay for preventive services, so the doctors wait for patients instead of trying to prevent illness and seek out those who need them most. Many heart patients present with serious illness after years of uncontrolled high blood pressure and other established risk factors such as obesity, smoking and high blood cholesterol levels. If their health insurance system had required an annual check-up, their doctor would have detected and controlled these risk factors earlier. This could contribute to the maintenance of health and avoid much distress and expense at the later stage.

It only needs one or two examples to show what, with hindsight, may be seen to amount to economic and social irresponsibility. Some governments are trying to catch up with a whole host of industrial diseases through their hospital and compensation services. Had there been priority for health, and proper consultation, industrial illnesses such as silicosis, pneumoconiosis, asbestosis, and cancers caused by toxic products would never have taken the toll they have. We do not know the cost of the widespread air pollution from power plants that have been built to keep pace with industrial demand. By inducing or aggravating respiratory diseases, they have undoubtedly caused enormous personal suffering and innumerable man-days lost to production. Many of these diseases are insidious in their development. Fifty years ago we had no idea of how many people were developing silicosis; thirty years ago we did not know that asbestos was so dangerous to health. Today, who knows how many people have impaired hearing because of high noise levels?

Viewed from this perspective, the situation shows gross financial mismanagement in terms of the cost-effectiveness of such industries, at the taxpayer's expense and at the cost of his health and that of his family. The environmentalists have been alerting society to the dangers of lead in petrol and other pollution from transport and industry, and they have persuaded public opinion to demand action in some cases. However, such action is usually at enormous cost, and much of the damage (and we only know the obvious bad effects) could and should have been avoided in the first place through proper coordination among ministries.

The problems of success. The proportion of elderly people in the European populations has been increasing steadily for the last 30 years. This success in extending life spans has brought new health problems: while the diseases of infancy and childhood have decreased, the more intractible diseases of old age have increased. Moreover, as the less-developed countries of the Region also become affluent the total size of the problem will grow, as the graph shows, at least until the end of the century.

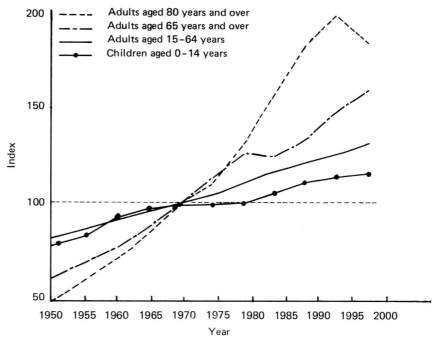

Source: World Health Organization (*7,8*).

Whose babies will die? In Europe in the last 30 years there has been a steady decline in the number of babies dying in their first year. There are still big differences, however, from country to country and between the rich and the poor in the same country. It is these differences which challenge our principles of equity and social justice.

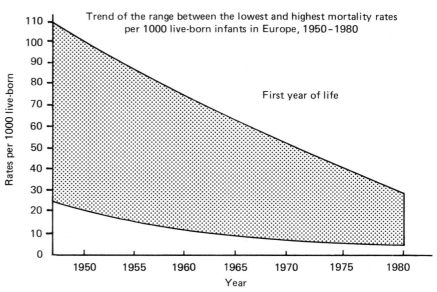

Source: World Health Organization (*7,8*).

Inequity

While there has been considerable progress in the health standards of the Region, it is obvious on looking back that far more could have been done within the resources available. There are still groups of the population who are grossly underserved and without effective access to health care. The major gap between the health standards of the different social or occupational groups has not been narrowed. For example, unskilled men are three times as likely as professional men to report chronic sickness (5); they are also much more likely to die earlier (6). Indeed, new problems are arising. The large numbers of unemployed young people throughout the European Region are almost certainly producing for that age group a new range of health problems associated with stress.

Although more and more people have gained access to social security schemes and health services throughout the Region, only in a minority of countries are all the people covered. Where social security systems exclude the more affluent section of the population, private health insurance generally fills the gap, but sometimes to the detriment of the public service. Health personnel may be attracted to the more remunerative private practice. There remain in some countries important minorities, such as the self-employed, small farmers, and their dependants, who are left out. There may also be inadequate provision for one-parent families, the unemployed, and immigrant workers who have not obtained sufficiently stable employment to gain access to social security systems.

Moreover, coverage by social security or a national health service does not in itself secure effective access. Travel costs, opening hours, loss of working time, costs falling directly on users, and cultural barriers may deter use. Even when a service is available, it may not be used in the best way because the people who need it do not know what problems should be taken where in the system. Usually the less well-off groups use services less than their state of health would warrant. For example, pregnancy may be notified to the services at too late a stage for adequate antenatal care. Services for infants and children, including immunization, may be grossly underused by poorer families.

Regional disparity

Throughout the Region services are biased towards hospital and specialist care at the expense of primary care. High-technology hospitals tend to be concentrated in the main cities. Where the primary care services are inadequate, hospital services tend to be used as costly and inappropriate substitutes. The socialist countries of the Region can claim with some justification to have succeeded in providing certain levels of health services to all the people. However, their success in

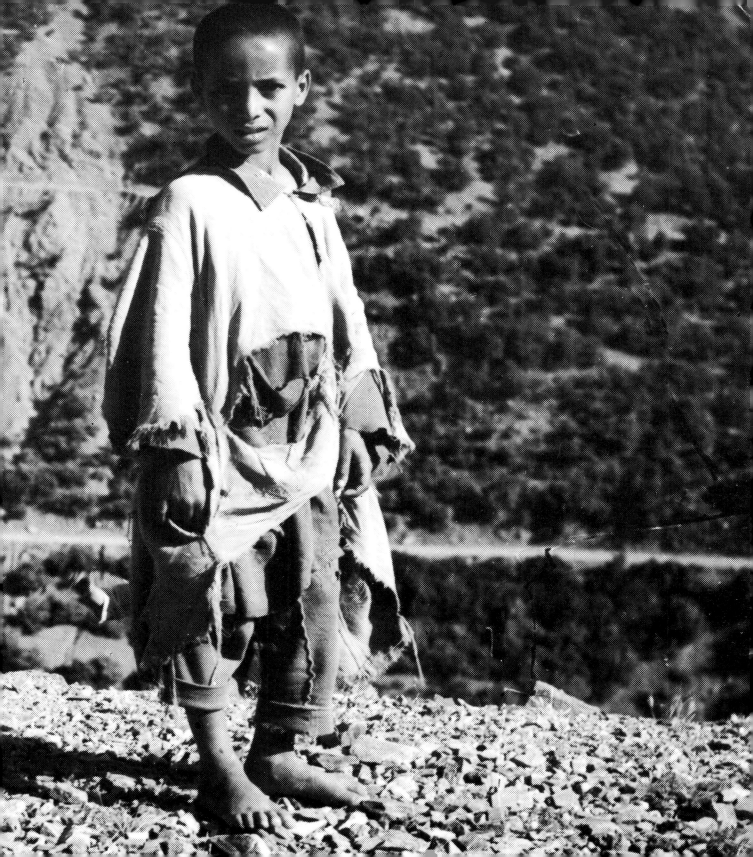

extending lifespans and their rapid industrialization have brought health problems, associated with aging and with stress due to the industrial environment and new lifestyles, which are similar to those of the other European countries.

In the wealthier countries of the Region progress has been uneven, and it hardly matches the enormous increase in resources. It may even be questioned how much credit for progress can be attributed to developments in the health care system. Among the more affluent nations there are countries with infant mortality rates as low as 8 per 1000, while others have rates twice as high. Some of these countries have maternal mortality rates as low as 5 per 100 000 live births, while others have three or four times as many maternal deaths. Mortality rates among the middle-aged (41–54) range from 370 to 720 per 100 000 of the population. These differences cannot be explained by levels of health spending, by the number of doctors and nurses or of hospital beds, or by any of the other usual health criteria. Generally, better health may have more to do with people having more money, better food, and better housing. Illness increases with recession, and the years since the Second World War have been mainly years of economic growth.

The paradox of poverty
Economic development has, however, often passed by the poorer areas of each country and of the Region as a whole. This poverty, in all its shapes and forms, remains the fundamental health problem of the European Region and indeed of the whole world. Most of the countries or areas which were poor 30 years ago are still poor today. Despite their valiant efforts it is impossible to expect people in such areas to pull themselves up by their own bootstraps.

Poverty, whether at national or international level, is not just children in rags, or tramps drinking raw alcohol. Poverty is a product of the way we run the whole of society. It is still endemic in Europe and it is still the biggest cause of ill health. Conversely sickness, like unemployment, is a significant cause of poverty. Hospitals will not remove poverty; they only cover its diseased patches until they break out in another place or form (5).

The later chapter on the cost of unemployment (page 137) deals with the way in which this classic form of poverty actually causes illness, and why we should do all we can to stop unemployment, even if only because it would save money. The problems of poverty run all the way through this book, and it is clear that health cannot just remain the province of a health minister who simply binds up the wounds of society.

Mortality by occupational class and age

Children (1–14 years)

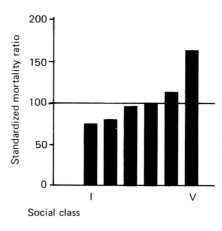

Adults (15–64 years)

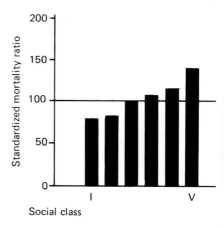

Source: Department of Health and Social Security (9).

Inequalities in health. Even in a "welfare state" with free health services more than twice as many children of unskilled labourers die before the age of 14 years as do children of professional workers.

It is a political and social problem of the first order. Poverty causes illness amongst pregnant mothers, their young children, their unemployed husbands. It aids and abets the effects of alcoholism, which are not just a damaged liver but include battered wives and babies. It makes education more difficult for the children and deprives them of prospects for the future. It causes more depression and suicide.

> The mother's psychiatric state and the presence of a serious long-term difficulty or a threatening life event were related to increased accident risk to children under 16. These factors were more common among working class children, and in so far as they are causal, they go a long way to explain the much greater risk of accidents to working class children. (*10*)

The industrial areas, however, even in recession, at least tend to benefit from a good structure of services for the local population, but there are still parts of the European Region that lack the basic requirements of pure water and effective sanitation. One of the most persistent sources of ill health is poor housing and sanitation. These conditions are bad enough when they affect families in stable communities, but they are even worse when they are added to the problems of the migrant worker or the immigrant. There are many pockets in the Region where overcrowded and inadequate housing is a major risk to health. A government policy of inaction to improve housing conditions because of "financial constraints" is probably short-sighted — the bill for ill health has to be paid in the end.

Even among unskilled adults the death rates remain nearly twice as high as those for professionals.

Problems of social change

The Region has been experiencing rapid social change. Some groups of people feel alienated from society, dissatisfied with current social institutions, and yet unsure of precisely what should be put in their place. The increased instability of the family creates insecure conditions for children and leaves some people in loneliness. The trend among women towards working outside the home has altered the role of the family as provider of care for children, the aged, and the disabled. Instead of expecting women to do at least two jobs, we should have expanded provisions for such social services as home help and nursery care to support them.

In the years following the Second World War there was a need for new housing and the immediate concern was to provide decent shelter for workers and their families whose homes had been destroyed or badly damaged. However, the planners produced vast impersonal new housing estates. Although the old cities were half destroyed or had outdated services they were still communities with a community spirit. The new estates became dormitories and little more. The planners made little or only belated provision for normal community or leisure activities and the first results were soon easy to see. Vandalism grew at alarming rates. This was, however, nothing like the wear and tear caused to the young mothers who peopled these estates, quite often without any support from grandparents who had preferred to remain in the decaying inner city areas. They were expected to take their children to shopping centres whose location had nothing to do with convenience for the young housewife. Bus fares were expensive and having done their shopping they then had to bring it and their children back home. Large numbers of people today live isolated lives in vast high-rise blocks or suburban estates, having little or no personal contact with their neighbours. More recently, similar problems have arisen for those left behind in rural communities as the exodus to the towns has depopulated the countryside.

In such a world of shifting moral and behavioural rules and collapsing social and economic barriers, people become more exposed and vulnerable because they have to rely more on themselves, lack guidance, and must take more responsibility for their own success or failure in the educational and social system. Social tensions can also arise, for example from the presence of underprivileged immigrant groups, especially if their ways of living are different from those of the rest of the population.

The elderly and change
For the elderly there are other difficulties. Those who did leave their old familiar surroundings often found themselves living in high-rise buildings, where they were even more deprived than young mothers, who at least had mobility and the physical resources to cope with difficulties. When vandalism struck, however, and the lifts went out of order the old were trapped, either literally or by the fear that they might have a heart attack if they tackled hundreds of stairs. The people living in such apartment blocks rarely met, except perhaps by chance in the lift — hardly the place for the development of community care. The planners found that they had razed a horizontal slum only to raise a vertical one. In addition, and particularly in the industrialized north of Europe, it has been becoming more and more acceptable — because of pressure on space, the cost of accommodation, the changing moral climate, the need to work — for families not to want to take responsibility for their needy members, whether young or old, or physically or mentally handicapped.

The mistakes of those planned housing deserts are now admitted but their effects are manifest in a whole generation. What is perhaps worse now, in social terms, is that the economic boom on which those housing estates were built has given way to a recession. The dormitory towns and housing estates were built for the boom years and depended on

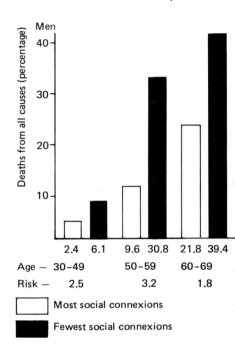

Social contacts and mortality

People need people. Isolation increases the risk of illness and death. People with "most social connexions" run a lower relative risk of dying than those with "fewest social connexions".

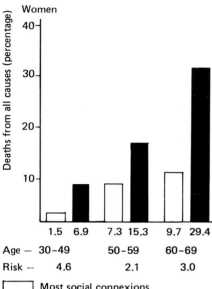

Source: Ferguson, T. (11).

It's worse for women. While women generally live longer than men, a lonely widow is three times as likely to die as her counterpart who still has companions, and socially isolated women in their thirties and forties may be four and a half times more at risk than those with friends.

the nearby factories. Now factory after factory is closing and the unemployment resulting is a new illness that is going to have many more effects than vandalism among those who have nothing to do except kill time. A pill, that most democratic tool of modern society, will not solve those problems.

UNBALANCED INVESTMENT

The rise in unemployment and the fear that it is going to stay high for the rest of the century at least have contributed to the chill wind that is blowing through society today. Another shock was the dramatic rise in oil prices in the early seventies, which coincided with a substantial fall in world economic growth. In an interdependent world the poorer developing countries have, in fact, been the hardest hit — just as the poor, unprotected groups in society feel the worst effects when social services are cut back because of recession.

If we are to find an overall health strategy that will work in this economic situation and be at least as good as and, it is to be hoped, much better than what we have now, we must look carefully at expenditure in the past. It is a fallacy to think that unlimited spending on high technology, even were it possible, is the road to a better system of health for all.

Some might think that the most painless way of attempting to achieve health for all would be to pour in extra resources in the hope that all the current gaps would be filled. This easy road is not economically feasible. Thirty years ago the more developed countries of the Region were devoting about 4% of their gross national product to health services. Today, health absorbs between 6% and 10% of their vastly increased resources. Because of the changed economic situation, the emphasis in many countries is now on containing health care costs, or at least on trying to prevent the growth rate from rising faster than that of the gross national product (12).

In many countries of the Region health expenditure has multiplied by several times in real terms within a span of only 25 years. General hospital beds have increased by 25%, nursing manpower by two thirds, and medical manpower has doubled. The share of resources consumed by acute hospital care and diagnostic services has been rising fastest of all. In terms of cost, hospitals now generally consume over half of national health budgets, and in some cases two thirds or more, yet hospitals cater for only a very small part of health needs. In the poorer countries the output of medical manpower has also increased substantially and there has been a rapid increase in expenditure on hospitals, particularly on teaching hospitals. Substantial research funds have been spent on the biomedical sciences, and companies throughout the world have invested enormous resources in the search for new drugs and for new medical equipment, but too little has been spent on trying to identify and prevent the fundamental causes of ill health.

While some action is being taken throughout the Region to improve the environment in which people live, work, and spend their leisure, there are still problems of gross pollution — particularly of rivers and of the sea. Air pollution has been reduced, although further improvement is still possible, and it could worsen again by the switch back to coal because of higher oil prices. Only in recent years has attention begun to be devoted to the problem of noise. The rapid introduction of new chemicals that affect air, water, food, and the working environment has posed new problems of identification of risk, surveillance, and control. The increasing use of nuclear energy involves potential risks from radiation hazards.

In the nineteenth century, although people gradually came to realize that contaminated water and poor sanitation were the cause of cholera and the other diseases that were decimating Europe, they were slow to respond and build the sewage and waterworks that were to reduce the death rates so dramatically. Now, in the late twentieth century, countries have been slow to find an effective response to the knowledge that the new diseases arising from lifestyles and the environment are having major effects on health.

Is this concrete jungle a home for the healthy? Housing authorities may be trying to provide homes for all by the year 2000 but this is not the environment that will help to achieve health for all.

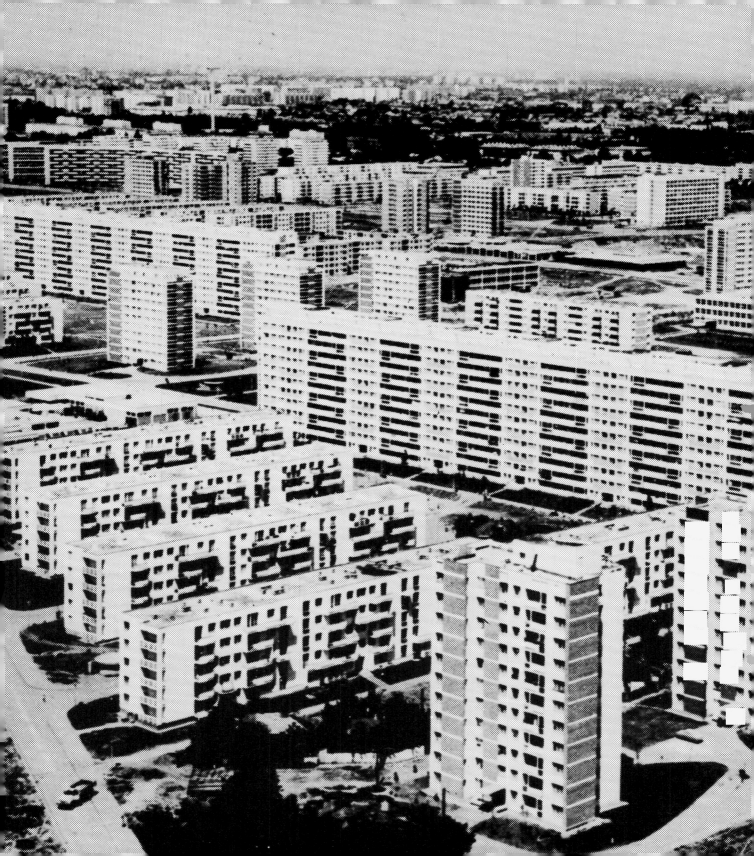

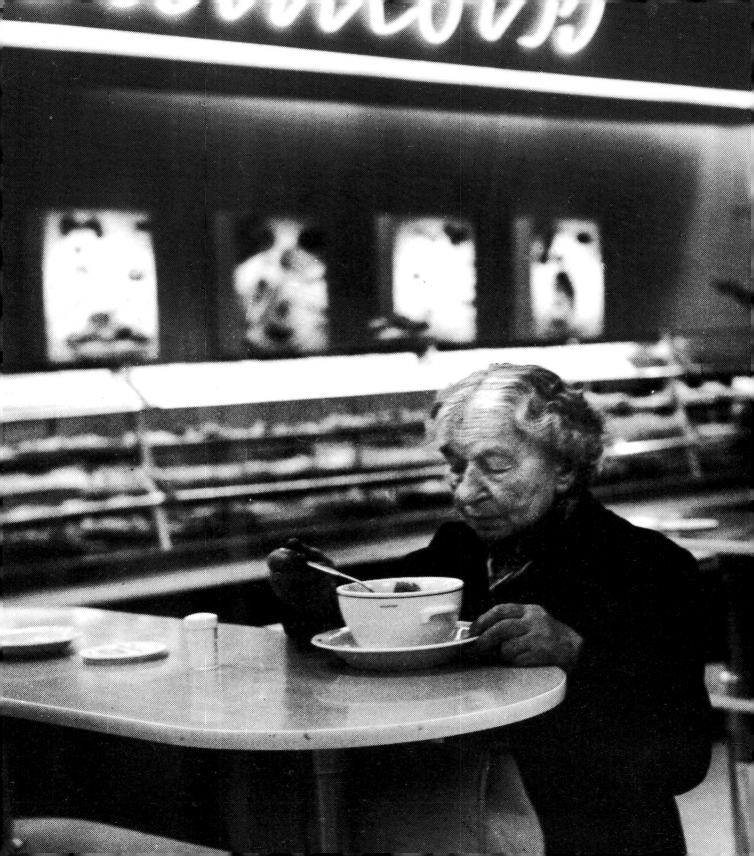

2.

The "New Diseases"

Plague, cholera, tuberculosis, diphtheria, scarlet fever, smallpox, typhoid — all are names that would have struck fear into anyone at the beginning of the century, yet in the minds of the majority of people in Europe today they count for little. Nevertheless, they are, in fact, much nearer home than many realize and, except for smallpox, have subsided only because a constant vigilance is maintained against them. Indeed, where it is not the disease may recur, as has happened with malaria in many parts of the world.

A more chilling realization is that, whereas the terrible afflictions of the past hold little dread, a host of "new diseases" has crept up on us and suddenly appears as the real threat to our future health. They are insidious in their approach and less obvious in their manifestations, so we know far less about their causes, although we are becoming daily more familiar with their effects. Those "diseases" include: cancer arising from environmental causes; deaths from smoking, alcoholism, and accidents on the road and at home; the abuse of medicines; drug addiction; mental illness; our neglect of the growing number of elderly people; and our general consignment of the responsibility for our own health to the professionals.

There has been pathetically little effort to tackle many of the factors behind these new diseases. What folly for a government to reap vast taxes for its exchequer from tobacco and alcohol only to have to spend as much, or more, on coping with their effects on health! Nor are the human misery and suffering, the social dislocation and unhappiness in families because of this induced illness remedied by government expenditure.

These diseases of affluent societies are also increasing in the less affluent countries of the Region. However, the less affluent countries still have a whole host of health problems which are now readily preventable by, for example, environmental or immunization programmes. Fortunately, the experience of the richer countries, which once themselves displayed a similar pattern of disease, may provide short cuts to better health for the less affluent.

THE NEW OUTCASTS

Many of the industrialized societies, which have much to learn from the poorer countries in the south of the Region, have made the tragic mistake of turning their elderly into a new deprived class. The old person is the new outcast of the twentieth century, an unproductive worker who must be kept at the least cost possible in an institution to await death. There is bitterness amongst the aged which often breaks through to the surface when they suffer contempt or ill treatment, and they demand to know why this is so. "Haven't I spent all my life working and paying my taxes; didn't I fight for my country . . .?"

The chronic diseases of old age creep up on all of us, however. In the majority of European countries mortality rates up to age 65 are low by world standards. Life expectancy at birth is between 65 and 73 years for men, and between 72 and 80 years for women. We have made life longer because of the advances in curative medicine, but we have done too little to cope with the problems of old age created by our success.

THE "NEW DEATHS"

As health standards improve, death rates alone become less relevant as indicators of a society's level of health; measures of disability, discomfort, and dissatisfaction become more important. Data using such measures are, however, not available for the Region as a whole, and such data as are available are based on varying definitions. The only complete and comparable information deals with deaths. This shows that diseases of the circulatory system account for more than half the deaths in 10 countries, and for more than 40% in 13 others. About 20% of all deaths are due to cancer, one third of them in the respiratory system. Although accidents cause only about 5% of all deaths, they are the largest single cause of death in children and young adults. About 10% of deaths are due to acute respiratory infections, pneumonia and influenza. In most countries the proportion of deaths primarily due to other infections and parasitic diseases is less than 2% (1).

DISEASES OF LIFESTYLE

Health problems due to lifestyle can be reduced by changes in behaviour, although changes will be difficult to achieve because the behaviour results from deep-seated cultural influences. Problems also result, however, from other factors that can be changed, such as the publicity given in the mass media to certain unhealthy habits and the sales promotion practices of manufacturers of products such as tobacco, alcohol, and baby foods, which directly affect health.

A failure to take regular physical exercise of the appropriate kind is seriously undermining health. Obesity and unbalanced nutrition are major problems in the more affluent countries of the Region, while lack of nutrients leads to stunted growth in the poorer countries.

It is worthwhile taking a look at some detailed analyses of these various "modern diseases" such as the overuse of medicines, alcoholism, other drug addictions, sexually transmitted diseases, smoking and some mental illnesses.

The pill-taking society

The over-use of drugs in the treatment of illness is a glaring example of the abuse of medicine — it is too often a palliative that fails to find the real cause and tackle it. The extent of this overuse is dramatically revealed in the statistics on the gap between the rich and poor nations of the world. The public health services of the 67 poorest developing countries, excluding China, spend less on all health care than the rich countries spend on tranquillizers alone. The answer, of course, is not for Europe to export more drugs, but to reduce its own consumption and collaborate with the Third World in supporting public health.

Alcohol for all

Experts have examined trends in alcohol drinking to find out on whom it was having the worst effect. Groups studied included young people, women, and immigrants, and also populations in developing countries. Evidence emerged not only that women, adolescents, and even young children were swelling the ranks of regular drinkers, but also that people were adopting a more "international" style of heavier overall consumption, over and above the traditionally established national patterns of drinking, such as taking alcohol with meals, drinking heavily at weekends, or indulging in extended drinking sessions. People were not only drinking the way they had done for years but had also begun to add the drinking habits of other nations: wine drinkers had taken to beer and spirits, and beer drinkers had learned that wine and their traditional brew were something they could mix.

The consumption of alcohol has increased considerably in most countries of the European Region over the last 25–30 years. In 1950 only France and Portugal had a consumption level of 10 litres per head per year. By 1975, ten countries were already over that level — two having increased their per capita consumption by more than 300% (2). More recent evidence indicates that France, at least, is now reducing its consumption of alcohol, but it still has a long way to go in this regard.

The international hard sell

Alcohol takes us into the realm of politics and commerce. Most important, perhaps, has been the internationalization of sales through the development of multinational corporations and cartels with powerful, almost monopoly, interests. Tourism, the international movement of labour, and advertising and the mass media have also had their effect on national and regional differences and, of course, on young people, who are the most exposed. Buying alcohol in off-licences and super-markets for home consumption has become socially more acceptable, and supermarket sales are growing fast.

There is recent evidence that certain groups of women may also be more at risk from adverse effects of alcohol. In Berlin in 1960 only 22% of alcoholics being treated were women, but in 1978 that figure had risen to 32% (2). There are various reasons for this, some of which are attributable to changes in social norms and lifestyles. Housebound women in late middle age, whose children have grown up and left home, are often lonely and isolated if their husbands are out at work all day. By middle age, spinsters and widows see themselves as leading aimless lives. With more spending power and greater social freedom, they take to drink as an easily available consolation.

The effect on the young is very clear. Surveys in Austria, the Federal Republic of Germany, and Portugal revealed that up to 80% of those aged 15 had already begun drinking. One of the most powerful fac-tors causing this was that young people wanted to seem more adult earlier; they copied their elders and had more money to buy drink. Moreover, the product itself was becoming cheaper in real terms and more easily available.

Alcohol in itself has a direct physical effect on the liver. When alcohol consumption is cut back nationally there is a dramatic change in the number of deaths from cirrhosis of the liver. The annual consumption fell by 10–20% in France in the 1940s and was accompanied by a 20% drop in deaths from cirrhosis. Delirium tremens was not seen in a Berlin psychiatric clinic during the Second World War, whereas in 1978, in a single day when a sample was taken, more than 200 patients had this condition (2).

Social escapism

The fact that society deceives itself can be seen in the way it defines drinking as a problem. It tends to look only at the obvious alco-holic — the person who makes a nuisance of himself and therefore stands out as having a problem. Anyone who drinks, however, may have a problem; to be suffering from the damaging effects of alcohol it is not necessary to be one of the 25–30% of people admitted to psychiatric hospitals in the Federal Republic of Germany and Ireland who, in fact, have drinking problems. One whisky before driving a car could result in death. A double gin at lunch and in the evening can easily become a growing habit and lead to alcoholism and cirrhosis.

Social attitudes have stopped us from collecting information to tackle this problem. Doctors have been too busy treating the physical effects, the police have been taking people to court (40% of all road accidents are associated with alcohol intake), social workers have been trying to help the families of heavy drinkers and protect the wives and children from beatings. Yet no one with decision-making powers seems to have set about taking the actions needed to prevent it all — least of all the governments who gain so much revenue from alcohol. That commerce and industry have not pushed harder for change because of the effect of drink on their profits and production is perhaps explained by the predilections of the managers themselves.

Alcohol is associated with cancer of the oesophagus, the mouth, and the larynx in spirit drinkers, and cancer of the large bowel in beer drinkers; it has known immediate and long-term effects on the nervous system; and it affects babies in the womb when pregnant women drink. This does not take into account broken limbs from falling down, accidents in front of cars or buses or with factory machinery, or pneumonia contracted after being drunk and out all night in the rain.

Various organizations in the Soviet Union have recently highlighted the problems connected with drinking and are deeply concerned about the enormous cost. Diseases caused by alcohol now rank third after heart disease and cancer throughout the Soviet Union. Heavy drinking is spreading rapidly among young people. Some 96% of young people begin drinking before the age of 18, usually spirits. The paper of the Communist Party's youth wing, *Komsomolskaya Pravda,* has reported that, in March 1980, 96% of people convicted of hooliganism were drunk, as were 68% of those convicted of aggravated murder, 67% of convicted rapists, and 57% of those convicted of inflicting bodily harm. Other Soviet surveys, covering the Georgian Republic, found that two thirds of alcoholics lived in cities, the majority were from broken homes and, although most had been treated for alcoholism, they had returned to drinking. Georgia, with a population of five million, spent a million roubles (about US $1 million) in trying to treat alcoholism. Industry lost more than 74 million roubles; 10% of all car accidents involved drinkers, and 12 000 people had their driving licences taken away for drunken driving. The social implications are no less disturbing; new housing estates have been terrorized by drunken hooligans who have smashed up cafés and cinemas and mugged people, including the old.

The national figures are as disturbing as these figures for Georgia. Bodies such as the Soviet Academy of Medicine are appalled at some of the effects, particularly the high percentage of mentally retarded children born to alcoholics. More and more children suffer because of growing

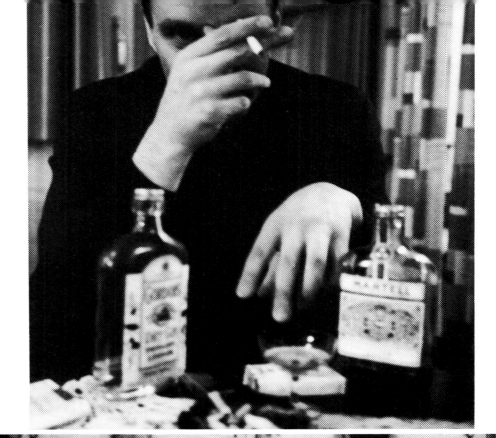

Drugging themselves to death. Many people who would not tolerate the use of "hard drugs" or even hashish consider alcohol as an everyday part of their lives. Yet this socially acceptable drug can be a killer. One drink before driving can lead to death. And it's not only the drunk who has a problem: the social cocktail can become a habit, leading to alcoholism, cirrhosis of the liver and death.

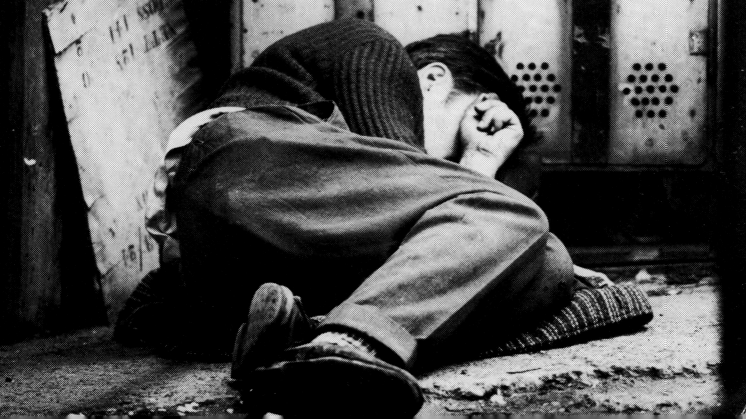

alcoholism amongst women, not only through damage to the foetus but also from later neglect, being badly fed, and living in an insecure and often violent home where the parents constantly quarrel. Many such children react later by taking to crime. In the Russian Soviet Republic, where about 50% of the total population of the Soviet Union lives, more than 50% of all fatal accidents in one year involved people who were drunk, and 25% of all accidents at work were caused by people with drinking problems.

The Soviet Union does well to keep such statistics: knowing the size of the problem is the first step to doing something about it. However, no country in Europe, big or small, is immune to the effects of alcoholism. Indeed, the fact that all countries have a problem in common suggests the urgent need for a common strategy to respond to it.

Narcotics — from Heaven to Hell
To the traditional drink as a means of drowning one's troubles younger people are adding narcotic drugs. Alcohol may kill in the long term, but the destructive effects of narcotics may come faster and may kill sooner. The process is quite horrific. It is true that the number of people on hard drugs is small compared with the number of those who damage themselves by smoking and drinking. The process of destruction of the young mind and body, however, is so fearful, and the rehabilitation process so long and difficult for the patient and for those helping, that it deserves special examination. The number of young people becoming addicted to hard drugs is growing and needs to be taken even more seriously than it is today.

Limiting and controlling the production of raw materials for drugs and placing a curb on trafficking are of great importance, nationally and internationally. However, most people turn to drugs because of pressures on their lives — the influence exerted by peer groups, lack of security, or poor employment prospects. The young people most at risk usually come from poorer backgrounds and from families with emotional and economic difficulties. The father and mother may drink, there is little love in the home, and often the child is pushed out of the house. Such children may do badly at school as a result and when they start dropping out they are quickly stigmatized as deviants. The things they often lack most of all, which are also often the key to their rehabilitation, are a sense of purpose in life and secure, stable relationships with other people, which do not need to come from parents, although for most of us that is the case. The child from the better-off part of society who becomes addicted has, of course, a better chance of rehabilitation because his family has better access to the support groups and services that are needed. Whether drug addiction afflicts the poor or the wealthy, however, the tragedy in human terms is the same.

Table 3. Europe: total consumption of alcohol (in litres of pure alcohol) per person aged 15 years and over[a]

An epidemic of alcoholism. For 25 years there has been a steady increase in the drinking of alcohol in almost all countries in Europe. Cirrhosis of the liver has shown an increase of epidemic proportions in the same time period. If the trend is not reversed, alcoholism will be one of the major killers of adults by the year 2000.

Country	1950	1960	1970	1979
Austria	6.5	11.2	15.8	14.3
Belgium	8.0	8.3	11.6	14.4
Czechoslovakia	5.3	7.5	10.9	13.5[b]
Denmark	4.9	5.6	8.8	12.2
Finland	2.4	2.6	5.7	8.1
France	22.1	23.4	20.5	20.5
German Democratic Republic	1.6	5.8	7.9	10.6[c]
Germany, Federal Republic of	3.8	8.7	13.5	16.0[b]
Hungary	6.4	8.3	11.5	15.7
Ireland	4.6	4.9	7.8	11.3
Italy	12.4	16.3	18.0	16.1
Luxembourg	8.5	10.5	12.9	16.8[c]
Netherlands	3.0	3.7	7.5	12.2
Norway	2.9	3.4	4.7	5.7
Poland	4.3	5.8	7.0	10.8
Portugal	—	15.3	16.3[d]	19.6[c]
Spain	—	11.6	14.9	19.6
Sweden	4.7	4.7	7.2	7.6
Switzerland	10.4	12.7	13.6	13.5
United Kingdom	6.3	6.6	8.4	10.3[b]
Yugoslavia	—	6.8	9.1	12.0[e]

[a] For each country, population data have been taken from the United Nations *Demographic yearbook* at the census year closest to the relevant year in the table.

[b] Estimate.

[c] 1976.

[d] 1972.

[e] 1975.

Source: Walsh, D. (*3*).

The road to hell starts with heaven. The drug pushers are a good example of users of market research and target consumer operation. They know how to use the free sample, what the market will take, when to hit it, and how to keep it hooked. They use that most successful promotion technique, pyramid selling: every new addict is a potential salesman because he will sell to others to get his percentage and so have enough money to buy for himself. Thus he will escape the horrors of deprivation and withdrawal. We fear the violence of the addict who mugs and even kills in his desperation to get money to satisfy his craving. Yet we fear nothing for what all this is doing to him as a person, mentally and physically. Instead, the "middle men" — the additional abusers, selling as well as using drugs — are the people who are picked up by the police and punished as "professional pushers". The big distributors are usually well protected by anonymity.

Once they are hooked, addicts who use a needle run the daily risk of infection and gradually destroy the veins in their arms and legs. Their life becomes a round of long bouts of intense craving followed by a few hours of relief. Any other interests they may have had become submerged. Their ability to use their skills, mental or physical, to get psychological reassurance from a personal relationship or to earn some kind of living is destroyed in the process, and they will rob and even kill to satisfy their craving.

Among drug addicts death often comes at an early age, ironically perhaps as a happy release from misery. It may be death by suicide, if not from illness or malnutrition. Addicts are at high risk of contracting many other illnesses, particularly as drug-taking is all too often associated with a "fix" in a dirty lavatory in a public place, or in a flat or house that is rarely cleaned. There is often no money left after buying the essential "fix" to buy even adequate amounts of food. The constant search for drugs leaves little time or inclination for cleaning up and the euphoric state makes the increasingly insanitary surroundings acceptable. Drug takers often combine their addiction with smoking and heavy drinking which makes their health even worse, and the risk is great that any children they have will be unhealthy and face a bleak future in a home that cannot hope to love and care for them.

Not all addicts "progress" inevitably to an early death. However, all too often when they do decide to try to stop, the clinic they go to cannot take them because it is full or running at half strength because of lack of funds. Society does not effectively support those working in this new and difficult field of rehabilitation. It refuses to have treatment centres in residential areas; it deprives them of adequate funds. The process of rehabilitation is costly, and report after report details how this or that

The slow slide down to hell. Although not all drug addicts "progress" inevitably to an early death, too many who seek treatment cannot find the support they need. A great deal of money is spent on law enforcement against drug trafficking while only a little is spent on preventing our vulnerable youth from becoming addicted in the first place.

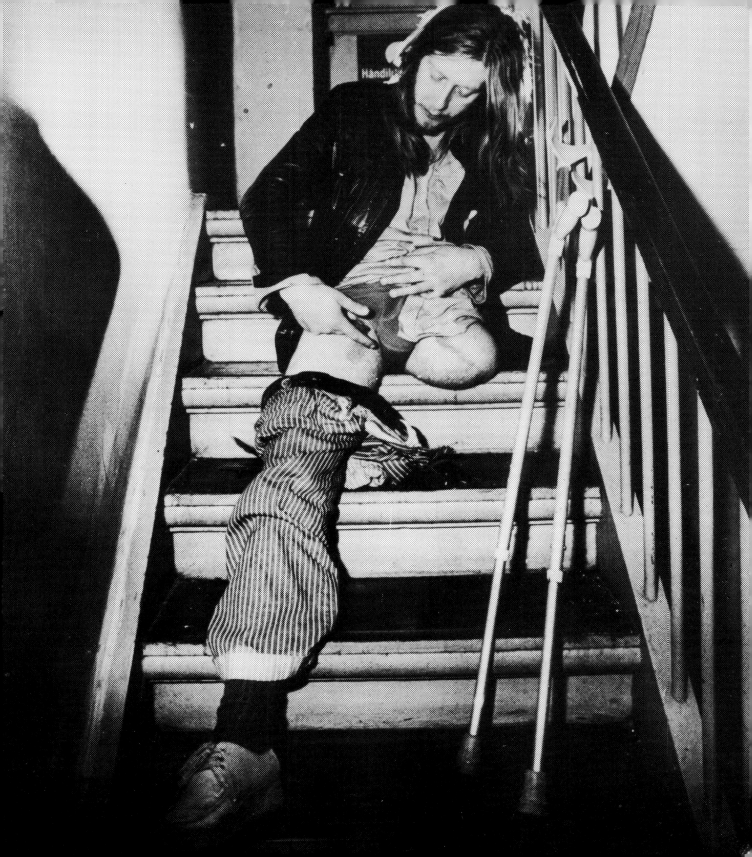

venture has been restricted or closed down for lack of public money. For those trying to help the addict the work is immensely tiring, both mentally and physically — they often wear themselves out trying to alleviate what appears to be a drive to self-destruction.

Unless there are major changes of policy, social attitudes, funding, and research into basic causes and treatment, several European countries will have a major problem by the middle of the 1980s. The tragedy is that the problem is already with us — not, as yet, in the shape of an overwhelming number of addicts but in our grave failure to recognize that the cause of the problem lies with society and society ought to be doing something.

Sexually transmitted diseases — the need for knowledge
A set of diseases that has long been with mankind — sexually transmitted diseases — has recently taken advantage of the dramatic movement of populations characteristic of the twentieth century. Advances in the field of drugs are very evident here because people affected with some of these diseases can now obtain quick and effective treatment — one penicillin injection is often enough to cure. Ironically, this makes prevention even more difficult. Because of the social implications and the secrecy with which society surrounds sexually transmitted diseases, the most essential part of prevention — follow-up and tracing contacts — is already not easy. The patient with an instant cure is now even less likely to collaborate. As a result, the particular microbe involved goes on to infect another person or mutates and spreads resistance to drugs which had previously been quite effective (4).

Moreover, many doctors are not alert to the wide range of sexually transmitted diseases and often know only the most common ones. Thus, cases that are simple to treat, such as herpes genitalis and mycoplasmal and chlamydial diseases, are often left to the individual to cope with, and can be a source of quite unnecessary pain and embarrassment. This is an example of the need for knowledge to be made more widely available, not only in the health profession but also among the public and particularly young people, who have been much more affected by these relatively uncommon diseases because of the changes in social habits and pressures.

Dying for a cigarette
People tend to think that the harmful effects of smoking are well known, but the figures show more than most people have realized. Smokers, men and women, die earlier than non-smokers, whatever the cigarette smoked. Some thought that they could switch from cigarettes to pipes, but that does not really work. Although the regular pipe smoker has a

higher risk than the non-smoker, it is true that because he does not inhale the smoke the risk is less than that for the cigarette smoker. The cigarette smoker who switches to pipes, however, may do nothing to decrease his risk because he will tend to continue inhaling smoke from habit. In fact, he may run a greater risk of dying from lung cancer or heart disease because he ends up inhaling the stronger smoke from pipe tobacco.

Eight out of every 10 people who die prematurely, die from smoking-related diseases: lung cancer, bronchitis and emphysema, various heart and circulatory diseases — not to mention cancer of the lip, tongue, mouth, larynx, pharynx, oesophagus, and bladder. Moreover, if you have a peptic ulcer and smoke, it will take longer to heal.

Tobacco deaths versus tobacco tax
In the United Kingdom it is estimated that about 25 000 deaths a year of people under 65 are directly due to cigarette smoking. In Sweden those aged between 35 and 85 have a 30–50% greater chance of dying early if they smoke. Every month in Sweden, out of a population of only 8 million, about 500 people die because they smoke. The more cigarettes an expectant mother smokes the less her child will weigh at birth. There is also a connexion between deaths in the womb and smoking mothers.

The smoking epidemic has spread dramatically. In Sweden the average number of cigarettes smoked annually per person aged 15 and over was 300 in the 1920s, 540 in the 1940s, 1360 in the 1960s, and 1610 between 1970 and 1975. A great deal more could be said on the indirect financial, social, and emotional cost of smoking, but it suffices here to mention a statistic from Sweden relating to 1970. In that year nearly 3200 people are known to have died as a result of smoking: 1700 from heart disease, 1200 from lung cancer, and 280 from chronic bronchitis. At the same time, 1100 people were turned into permanent invalids as a result of their smoking habits (5). The total economic loss was estimated at 1100 million Swedish kronor (more than US $250 million at 1977 prices). That figure includes 200 million Swedish kronor in nursing costs and 900 million in lost production. It also represents nearly half the Swedish Government's revenue from tobacco. The cost in human suffering remains uncounted.

There are one or two other, less obvious but perhaps more disturbing, side effects of smoking. Wheezing is more common in children up to the age of five if the parents smoke. The risk of a young child developing bronchitis in the first year of its life is doubled if its parents smoke and the child inhales the smoke from the air in the home. If the parents cough and produce phlegm dispersed as droplets in the air the risk is

Lighten up!
Share today's light Belair!

Only one low 'tar' tastes Belair fresh.

BELAIR

Kings & 100's

LIGHT MENTHOL · LOW TAR

Numbers of cigarettes smoked per adult per year

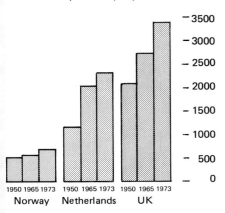

1950 1965 1973 1950 1965 1973 1950 1965 1973
Norway   Netherlands   UK

Lung cancer deaths per 100 000 population

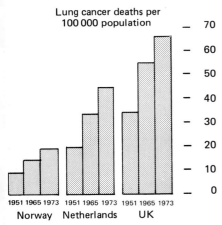

1951 1965 1973 1951 1965 1973 1951 1965 1973
Norway   Netherlands   UK

Tobacco is a killer. The rise in cigarette smoking throughout Europe is paralleled by the rise in lung cancer. The countries with the highest rate of cigarette consumption also have the highest rate for cancer deaths.

Deadly seduction. Millions are spent on advertising, often using implicit or even overt "healthy" sporting and sexually enticing images, which lures thousands to an early death and adds a huge burden to the cost of health care.

Table 4. More cigarettes: more cancer

Country	Manufactured cigarette consumption[a] per adult per annum[b]				Lung cancer deaths per 100 000 population[c]		
	1935 (no.)	1950 (no.)	1965 (no.)	1973 (no.)	1951	1965	1973
Austria	860	1100	1930	2550	30	41.7	43.3
Belgium	790	1240	1980	2730	—	39[d]	51.3
Denmark	470	1290	1500	1850	13.2	31.2	40.4
Finland	1350	1640	1920	2040	21.8	32.3	38.1
France	530	930	1510	1920	17.5	20.4	25.4
Germany, Fed. Rep. of	—	630	2100	2610	16.7	31.8	35.6
Greece	960	1600	1930	2550	—	21.1	30.8
Iceland	480	1490	1840	2030	—	—	11.8
Ireland	1210	2510	2690	3340	12.9	—	—
Italy	450[e]	660[f]	1540	1930	9.7	19.9	30.1
Netherlands	680	1120	2020	2370	18.5	32.4	44.3
Norway	300	510	520	640	7.4	11.7	18.4
Portugal	270[g]	620	1130	1490[h]	—	6.4	10.5
Spain	390	430	1760	2260	—	—	17.2
Sweden	380	810	1360	1580	9.2	16.3	24.6
Switzerland	540[i]	1500	3050	3370	19	23.8	32.2
United Kingdom	1590	2180	2680	3230	33.5	55.3	65.4

[a] The consumption per adult per annum figures are based on the total sales of tobacco goods and the population aged 15 years and over resident in each country. In some countries, notably Switzerland, the consumption per adult statistics are exaggerated due to the appreciable volume of sales to borderers, tourists and seasonal workers.

[b] *Source:* Tobacco Research Council (*6*).

[c] *Source:* World Health Organization (*7,9*).

[d] Figures are for year 1952.

[e] Annual average, year ended 30 June 1931 — year ended 30 June 1935.

[f] Annual average, year ended 30 June 1946 — year ended 30 June 1950.

[g] Figures are for year 1940.

[h] Figures are for year 1972.

[i] Annual average 1934–1937.

even greater for the children. More frightening is what we do *not* know about the effects of smoking because not enough research has been done. Some recent studies suggest that cigarette smoke may cause genetic changes which will be passed from parents to children, and that congenital malformations may occur in children whose parents smoke. One survey has shown a 28% increase in deaths at the time of birth when the mother smoked. This could be due to the effect of the carbon monoxide in cigarette smoke, which reduces the oxygen-carrying capacity of the blood; babies in the womb thus have their oxygen supplies cut off by their smoking mother.

THE MENTALLY ILL – PRISONERS OF MIND AND BODY

Mention was made above of the old person as an outcast in modern society, particularly in the industrialized world. The darker side to that rejection by society concerns the mentally ill, many of whom have either grown old in mental institutions or entered them at an advanced age. There have been, fortunately, radical changes from the barbaric treatment that was once meted out to those who did not fit into the community, but society still stands guilty of shutting away the problem instead of seeing it for what it is: an extension of the pressures and difficulties that are produced by society, quite often as capable of treatment as any other deficiency in health. Because of social changes in certain Mediterranean countries, too, a growing number of children there are showing symptoms of psychiatric disturbance. Isolation in an institution for the mentally disturbed may have been the common reaction in industrialized societies for the past two hundred years, but it is a form of treatment that must be radically rethought. The scale of the problem can be gauged from statistical estimates of the number of mentally ill people in the world today – 40 million, approximately the population of Spain and Portugal. They are often the product of an unthinking society that has turned more refugees onto the roads because of political and military conflict since the turn of the century than the world has ever known. However, it is not just wars that have destroyed the stability of communities; the migration of populations in search of work, the stresses of urbanization, the effects of drugs and alcohol, all take their toll and boost the numbers of mentally ill.

There are still more than one million people in mental hospitals in the European Region and a quarter of these establishments have more than a thousand beds, making them too large and unwieldy (8). The result is usually impersonal prison-type regimes where there is little privacy and no stimulus to the development of intellectual abilities or social contact.

Out of sight, out of mind. There are still more than one million people in mental hospitals in Europe. A quarter of such hospitals have more than a thousand beds, with prison-type regimes, little privacy and none of the stimulus and social contact that people need to help them get better and return to society.

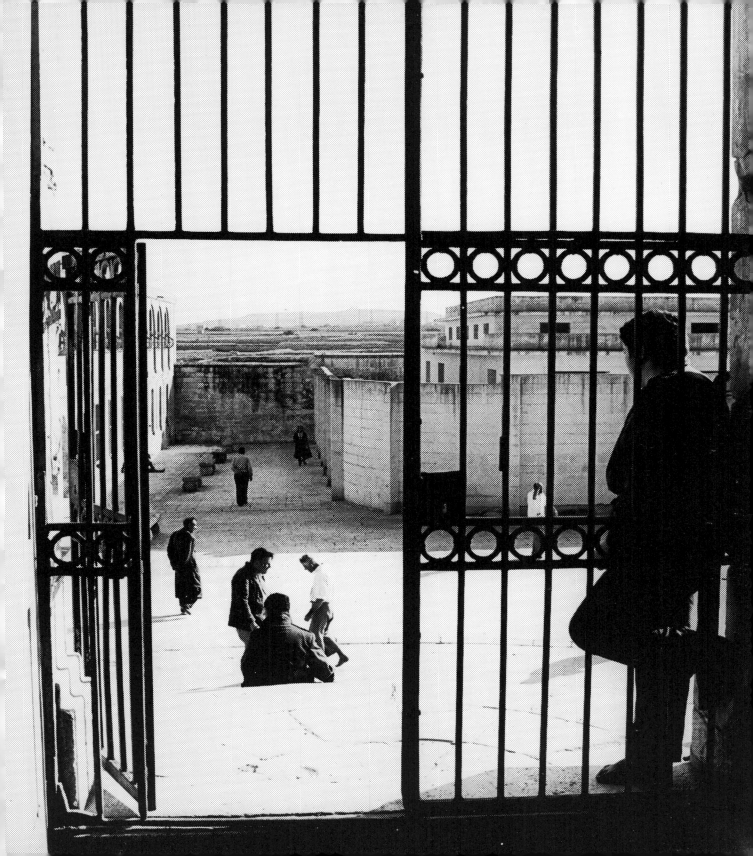

Table 5. Suicide and self-inflicted injuries, 1950 and 1975: rates per 100 000 total population[a]

Country	1950	1975
Austria	23.8	24.1
Belgium	13.1 (1952)	16.2
Bulgaria	7.4 (1953)	12.9
Czechoslovakia	—	21.9
Denmark	23.3	24.1
Finland	15.6	25.1 (1974)
France	15.2	15.4 (1970)
German Dem. Rep.	—	30.5 (1970)
Germany, Fed. Rep. of	19.8 (Berlin (West), 1951)	20.9
Greece	3.6 (1955)	2.8
Hungary	17.8 (1954)	38.4
Iceland	11.9	10.1
Ireland	2.6	5.0
Italy	6.5	5.8 (1972)
Luxembourg	11.0 (1951)	10.6
Malta	14.9[b] (1952)	0.6 (1973)
Netherlands	5.5	8.9
Norway	7.4	9.9
Poland	5.4 (1954)	11.4
Portugal	10.0	8.5
Romania	—	59.9[c] (1974)
Spain	5.4	4.0 (1974)
Sweden	14.9	19.4
Switzerland	23.5	22.0
Turkey	0.4 (provincial capitals)	0.3 (provincial capitals)
USSR	—	—
United Kingdom	9.5	7.8 (England & Wales, 1974)
Yugoslavia	55.3[d] (1952)	13.4

[a] Rates are based on the populations of each country at the census year closest to the relevant year in the table.

[b] This figure includes All Other Accidents, Suicide and Self-inflicted Injuries.

[c] This figure includes All Other Accidents, Suicide and Self-inflicted Injuries, All Other External Causes.

[d] This figure includes Motor Vehicle Accidents, All Other Accidents, Suicide and Self-inflicted Injuries.

Source: Walsh, D. (*3*).

Unnecessary deaths. In the majority of European countries the suicide rate is increasing, all too often claiming the lives of young people. Yet research into the causes of these tragic deaths is rare.

Yet it is just such stimulus and contact that are essential to rehabilitation and return to the community. The rapid advance of medical technology and the increased demand for medical services of all kinds have also contributed to the spread of impersonal care.

Throughout the Region alcoholism has produced severe mental problems, yet no country seems to have mounted an effective programme against it. In Europe as a whole, too, mental health information systems are non-existent, rudimentary or, at best, only modestly developed.

100 000 suicides a year
More than 100 000 suicides occur in Europe every year. Alcohol and other drugs have compounded the problem of suicide, which is one of the major causes of death among young people. Yet society turns a blind eye to the death of young people in this manner.

Most governments spend too little money on their mental health services, and treat them in the same way as society does — as a necessary evil on which the less spent the better. "Out of sight, out of mind" has the makings of a pun too cruelly near the truth. The neglect of research in this field, in comparison, say, with market research into the kinds of dog food people prefer to buy, can be seen from one of the few intercountry studies undertaken (in 1976). WHO sent a questionnaire to its Member States, but the study was severely hampered by the countries' inability to give any useful detail in answer to the questions. It seemed that nobody had really bothered to keep the kind of statistics needed.

The hostile institution
One danger of specialized psychiatric care is that it puts people who need community care into a hostile institutional environment. Mental institutions progressively institutionalize their residents and alienate them more and more from society. Several countries still have laws making entry into an institution compulsory in certain cases and allowing treatment to be carried out against a patient's will — quite often without the knowledge of relatives. Such laws and practices may obscure understanding of the issues involved. Elderly people who are mentally ill are patients needing special care, and the greater our lifespans the more needs of this kind will grow. In some countries almost half the beds in mental hospitals are occupied by people over the age of 65, often because there is a shortage of suitable accommodation and care in ordinary hospitals.

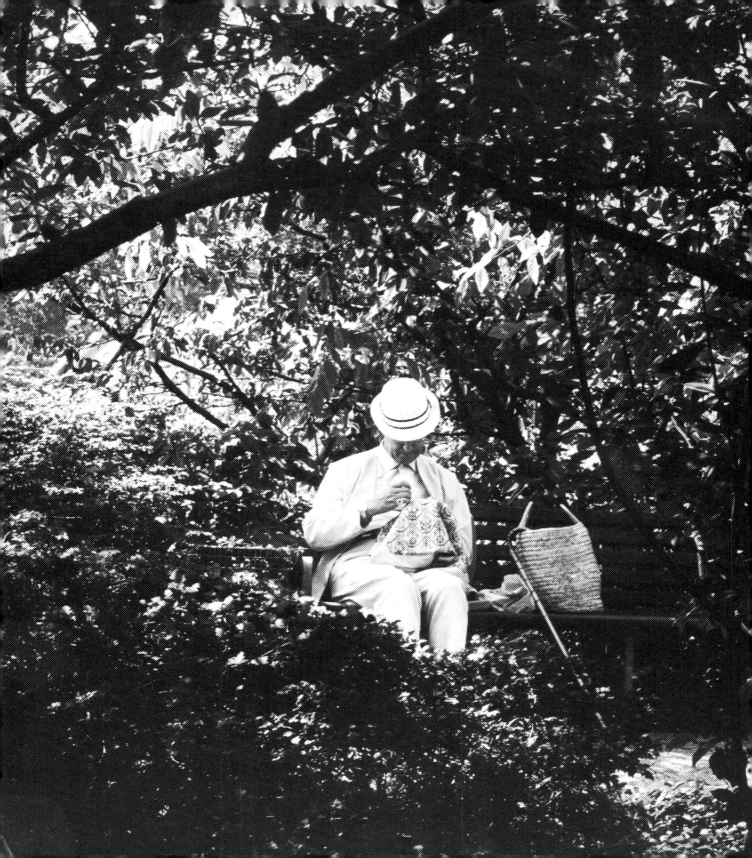

3.

Loss of caring
in the community

THE TEAR AND REPAIR SOCIETY

The affluent industrialized society has, in a way, sown the seeds of its own destruction. The attitudes of built-in obsolescence, that you "can always get another one", have spilled over into the realm of personal health. People have come to assume that they can abuse their bodies as much as they want and the medical services will repair the damage. Even if there is no miracle cure, they feel that one will certainly be discovered in due course. Those ministries which have ignored the importance of health in their plans for industrial development are equally guilty of this approach. The wonders of spare-part surgery, however, are no substitute for taking steps to see that the spare parts are not needed in the first place; the advent of heart transplants means that those with transplants are daily living with death. The fact that the risk of this kind of operation is justified in some cases is not a reason for living a life that risks creating the condition for which the operation is needed. It would seem almost that society manufactures illness as a product it distributes, so that it can then move along to stage two — after-sales service.

Our society in the European Region is one that overeats to the detriment of bodily function, and then wastes time, money and effort trying to lose weight. The moral aspect of that situation in the light of the hunger existing in the world needs little emphasis, yet people fail even to see the economic stupidity of it in relation to their own purses.

Willing prisoners of the medical profession

Having inflicted wounds on ourselves, in one way or another, we turn to the repairers to see what they can do for us. Our pursuit of the advantages that the new drug and technology revolution can offer has produced the most amazing effects when it comes to the service we get from the medical profession. Because self-care has become so little a part of our approach to health, we find that some medical personnel, from the lowest ranks to the often remote and rarely seen consultant, tend to look down on the patient from the Olympian heights of their professional mystique and knowledge. Some display an attitude of benevolent paternalism towards the patient. Fortunately this is not true of the whole of the profession, but there is quite sufficient of this attitude to make it a cause for serious concern (1).

The Director-General of WHO has hard words for the medical profession in the context of pressing global health problems:

> Any thoughtful observer of medical schools will be troubled by the regularity
> with which the educational system of these schools is isolated from the health

A prisoner of the medical profession. Prodded and poked by a galaxy of experts, a child is helpless in the medical maze

service systems of the countries concerned. In many countries these schools and faculties are, indeed, the proverbial ivory towers. They prepare their students for certain high, obscure, ill-defined, and allegedly international "academic standards" and for dimly perceived requirements of the twenty-first century, largely forgetting or even ignoring the pressing health needs of today's and tomorrow's society.

Most of the world's medical schools prepare doctors not to care for the health of the people but to engage in a medical practice that is blind to anything but disease and the technology for dealing with it. Sometimes even the cynical question is raised: does it really matter what kind of doctors we train? (2)

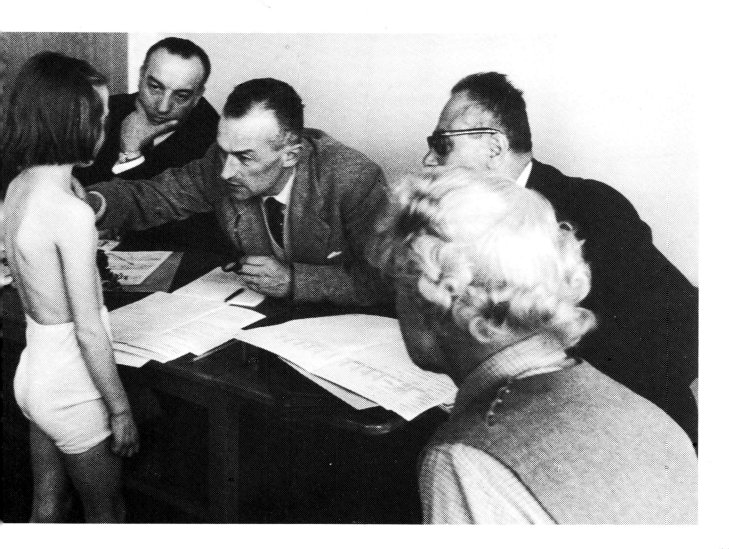

The medical maze

For many patients the local doctor is the first step into a world of mazes and corridors. Patients in any case often consult more than one doctor for the same episode of illness or, for different episodes, different doctors chosen according to the specialty the patients think appropriate. Many patients do not have a personal doctor, let alone a family doctor, to provide continuity of care based on a knowledge of their past medical history. In some systems of medical care not all the specialists have access to hospital beds, and not all hospital specialists have outpatient clinics. Thus, a patient may be referred from a community-based specialist to a hospital-based specialist. Both specialists may undertake similar diagnostic tests, an added burden on the patient and on the social security system that pays the cost of both.

Where primary care services are inadequate, hospital services tend to be used as costly and inappropriate substitutes. Health care in hospitals is often criticized as being dehumanizing and unduly technical; patients feel that they are treated like objects, inadequately informed, and given no opportunity to discuss their treatment. If there is a local doctor, he often has had no adequate refresher training since he graduated, and he may still be working on his own or with a colleague of his own age. Many doctors work well beyond a retirement age that would not be allowed in other professions with such responsibilities. Local doctors, in contrast to the overspecialization of their hospital colleagues, often seem to avoid using many of the cheap, modern techniques for testing which are now available and which could save their patients from going to a hospital for routine tests.

In a sense the public has made itself a prisoner of the medical profession. The latter jealously guards the right, in most countries, to try its own members for professional negligence. It decides on the amount of information it will impart to the very person who is the whole justification for the profession, the patient himself. This attitude may have been valid, and even perhaps wise, before the advent of universal education, but members of the medical profession have often failed to move with the times when it comes to responsibility to the patient. It has also had the effect of making too many people assume that health means cure and that the only person who can achieve that cure is the doctor. This has turned many doctors into work-horses and deprived their patients of much of their real skill and knowledge as they have tried to cope with overburdened practices.

Safe, but not comfortable
Health care in hospitals is often
dehumanizing and unduly
technical, so a person feels trapped
among wire and machines

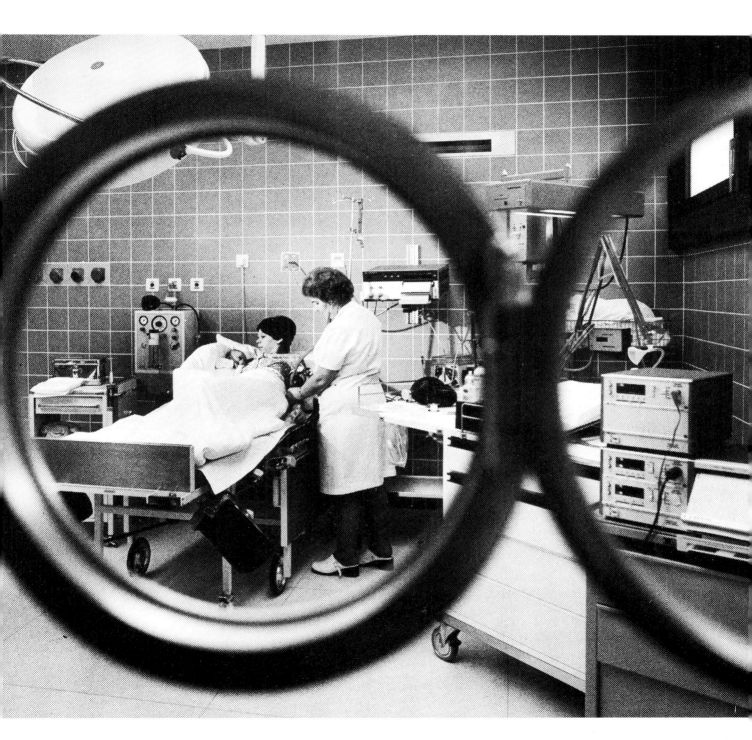

COMMUNITY CARE

It is this mystique imparted to the role of the medical worker, of whatever rank, that brings us finally to the greatest self-inflicted loss of all — the loss of a caring community, the loss of the once widely-held belief that looking after yourself and your own was the first role of the individual, the family, and the community. There is a stark contrast between the massive and amazingly complex life support systems that today cater for the patient undergoing open heart surgery and the horse-and-buggy physician with his little black bag who represented primary medical care at the turn of the century. Yet it is this stark contrast which is at the root of the problem that most of Europe faces today. We have moved far away from that concept of primary health or community care. We have made many gains but have lost the lessons of centuries.

During the history of medicine primary medical care has been by far the most important approach to providing health services. The horse-and-buggy physician and his predecessors through the ages were clearly practitioners of primary medical care. With all our modern advances, however, the hospital became the natural workshop of the doctor. The value of primary health care, which could have kept many people out of hospital, was more and more ignored, and the result was the neglect of their health. There is no doubt that the developed world, as it sees newly designed schemes being brought forward in the developing countries, has become more aware of the need to move back to community care. There is much to be learnt from the long traditions of community care in those countries as well as from the new schemes.

The hospital in the late 1950s was responsible for doing a lot of damage to the real promotion of health (3). It was seen as the provider of life-blood for all the health services. The services would radiate out from the hospital, supposedly reaching everyone. We now know that hospitals cannot provide that kind of comprehensive service and, in fact, are responsible for only a tiny fraction of health services. If we look back over the whole spectrum of developments in public health during this century we can see that, particularly amongst the medical profession, health has been misunderstood as being a matter of hospital-based medicine and specialization. Those who make a living out of disease get more emotional and intellectual satisfaction from specialized care than from primary care, which seldom offers the drama and public acclaim of major surgery. The public is not blameless in this matter either. It has demanded sophisticated high technology, looked down

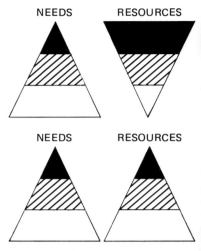

Balanced needs and resources

■ Specialist care

▨ General hospital care

☐ Primary health care

Balancing resources and needs requires a complete inversion of the present health systems. At the moment they have inadequate resources for prevention among the community and concentrate their main expenditure on specialist use of costly high technology. Shift resources from the top to the bottom of the pyramid and primary health care needs will be better met, people will remain healthier and the demand for specialist care will be reduced.

What is health? It is not merely the absence of illness. It is the enjoyment of all those faculties which we possess as individuals. Even the most severely handicapped can enjoy life by their own standards

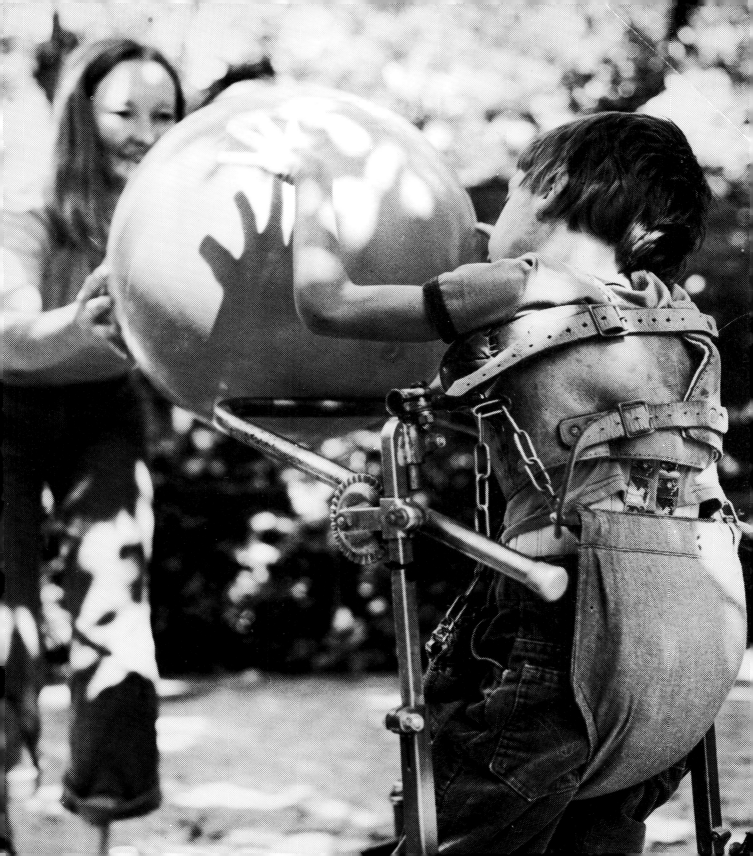

its nose at primary health care, and all too often equated "primary" with "primitive". This attitude did not just materialize out of thin air; the public in effect adopted the prejudices of the medical profession. However, the damage had been done in effectively turning local and primary services, as well as self-care, into some kind of weak, poorly organized, bedraggled Cinderella.

In the remainder of this book the aim will be to outline the response that the World Health Organization proposes to the problems we have allowed to mushroom. The two most important groups of people who are going to make that response are the public and the medical profession. Without that involvement there is no hope of rediscovering community care. With it we shall have begun one of the most important social changes that society will see in the second half of the twentieth century.

THE LESSONS

The first essential is that individuals and society regain control over their own health through a full acceptance of their own duties and responsibilities. The second is to change fundamentally the way we treat the illnesses that afflict modern society — illnesses that, in fact, it mostly inflicts upon itself. Most of these are preventable illnesses, and so another essential strategy must be to identify them, evaluate them, and take action against them.

WHO believes that this new appraisal of the health of nations is as valid for developed as for developing countries, for industrialized as for rural societies. The WHO Regional Office for Europe has been working for the past three years with experts from its Member States to define the basic principles of a detailed new health scheme for all 33 countries in the Region. This is a job it has been doing, along with other WHO regions, since the Alma-Ata International Conference on Primary Health Care ended in September 1978. No scheme involving the individual can be imposed from above. The strategic framework spelt out in the rest of this book is an outline of the basic principles for action. These principles require adaptation to each national cultural environment, but they will grow in strength as each country in the Region "fleshes them out". There is great strength in unity through diversity, and as research develops throughout the Region so unity of purpose will emerge. It is this unity which is required if the people of the European Region, from Iceland to Morocco, from Dublin to Vladivostok, are to reach the year 2000 with the prospect of health for all.

. . . the healthy handicapped need due consideration, however, when society is designing the everyday facilities that all of us need to use.

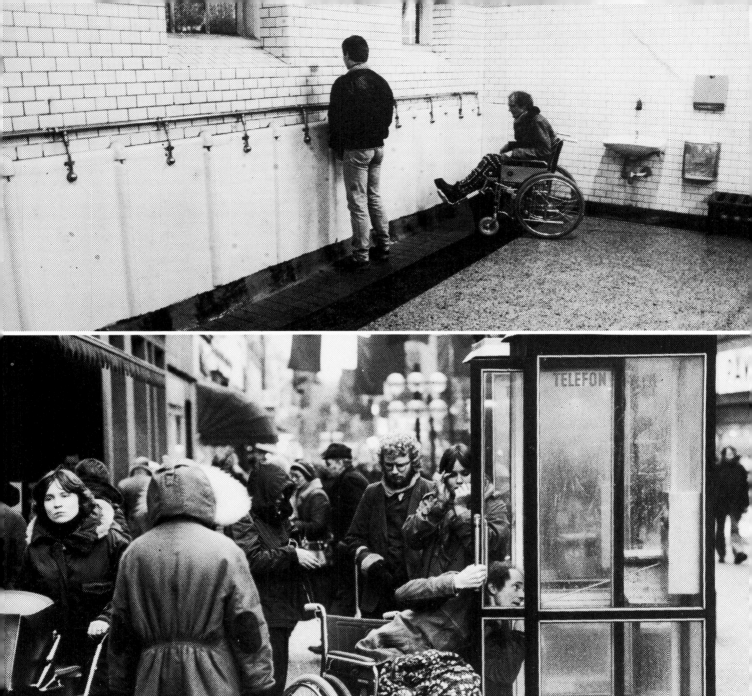

FINDING AN ANSWER — THE STRATEGY

The Strategy for Attaining Health for All by the Year 2000 will fail unless we succeed in moving the pendulum back from the misuse of high-technology, hospital-based health services. Health is primarily a matter of self-care. If that approach is to permeate our society we must harness the support of individuals, families, and health professions by inculcating a philosophy of primary health care. A more personal title, which reveals the foundation on which it must rest to succeed — the caring community — is community care.

What is health?

Health is not merely the absence of illness. It is the enjoyment of all those faculties which we possess as individuals. We consider later how the elderly and the mentally ill, examples of the weakest groups in our society, can be given a full social role. By implication the same principles apply, even though they will not be spelt out, to the physically handicapped and those suffering from visual impairment or even total blindness. These are "weak groups" only because we regard them as such. These groups are often stopped by the rest of us from helping themselves. They are the specialists in their needs, yet we do not ask them about or involve them in the things we do. There is no one more frustrated than a person in a wheelchair trying to use a telephone box which even an able-bodied person sometimes has difficulty getting into, never mind then trying to reach the 'phone receiver! The classic case is of the architect who, if he remembers at all, decides that chairbound people should be able to get about in his new building. He installs automatic doors at street level with no step, but forgets to place the lift buttons within reach of a person who is seated. How many chairbound people does he actually call in for advice? These groups have their own networks that we should call on. By getting old people to manage themselves and giving them the environment to do so at home, making their kitchens a little safer or designing easy-to-hold pans for arthritic hands, we are actually helping them to stay healthier. We also help to keep them out of hospitals, where they would often just fade away. In Luxembourg the postman actually has the job of knocking on the doors of elderly people every day to ensure that they are all right. That is community participation. (4)

This participation emerges throughout the stages of life from birth to death. Each stage has its limitations imposed by nature, which determine the responsibilities, needs, and rights of each age group. In such a framework the community will care for itself. Thus, the adults of society, both male and female, must shoulder the burden of looking after the young, the sick, the handicapped, and the elderly — and they, in their turn, will be provided for. When society accepts this framework it will enjoy the certainty and security of community care.

The Strategy's three themes
There are three overlapping themes in the Strategy, which form its core and must be given substance by different groups and nations:

- health as a way of life,

- the prevention of ill health,

- community care.

The promotion of health, through education or information, is inextricably bound up with every response or plan we devise in these three areas. In one sense there are no special groups in our society. We are all special groups with varying needs at varying times according to the stage of life through which we are passing.

Change involves us all
The Strategy must be put into effect by individuals in and through their communities, and by those who work in the health professions. We must get everyone to look at his particular job in life and see the health element involved: from the engineer who designs sewage systems for housing estates to the microchip designer. The same applies to environmental lobbyists, civil servants, politicians, and organized groups such as the blind. How the necessary changes can be made by the community at large, and the new challenge that this involves for the health profession, are discussed in some detail in the two sections which follow.

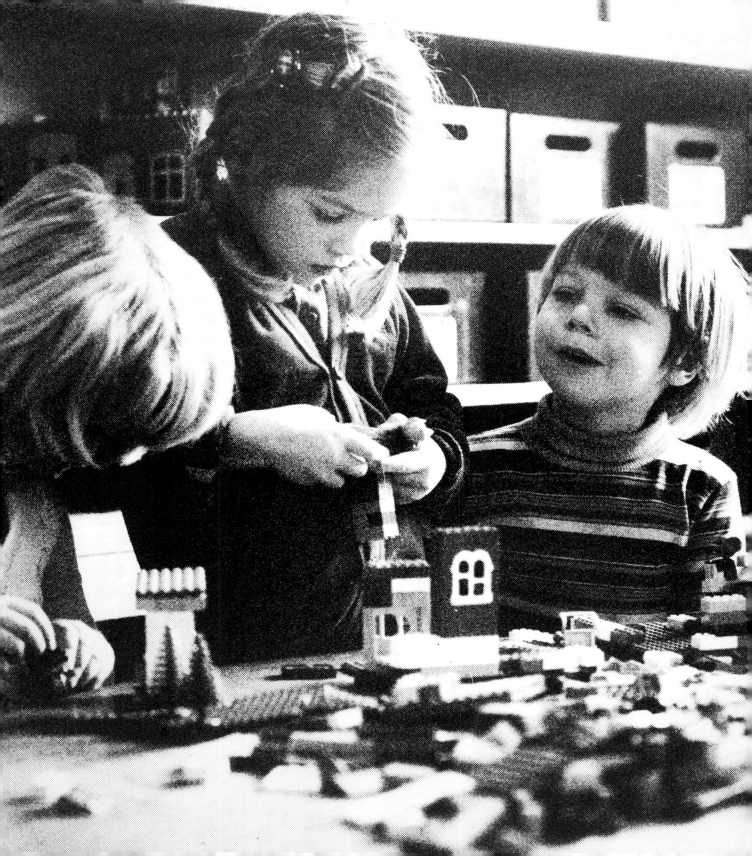

4.

Self-care and consumer participation

We come now to the most challenging part of our work, namely the inability of most health services to respond properly to the needs of communities. We often refer to "coverage" by the health services and, with obvious pride, we say that such and such a facility has been established to cover such and such an area where so many thousands of people live. We do not seem to realize that coverage, to be valid, must relate to productive contact between the health service and people for specific needs . . . The reality is that, of the people to whom the facility is said to be available, only the minority who live closest to it actually use it. The majority are excluded . . .

But a simple extension of conventional health services, no matter how far-reaching into the community, is unlikely to produce the necessary improvement. Health is not a commodity that is given. It must be generated from within. Similarly, health action cannot and should not be an effort imposed from outside and foreign to the people; rather it must be a response of the community to problems that the people in that community perceive, carried out in a way that is acceptable to them and properly supported by an adequate infrastructure.

The spirit of self-reliance — at the individual level, the family level, the community level and the national level — will be fundamental to any strategy for achieving health for all. Self-reliance sets people free to develop their own destiny. It is the essence of primary health care. *Halfdan Mahler (1)*

Roles of the individual and the family

In ensuring good health the most important person is the individual. Self-care, and self-management where there is a chronic condition, should not be regarded in the traditional sense of certain do's and don'ts drummed into a person by everyone from the school nurse onwards. It means an awareness that a healthy life is a matter of one's job, housing conditions, food and lifestyle, not just avoidance of the risk of catching something.

The family can adopt the same self-care role on a sharing basis. The family is perhaps the most powerful educational element in any society and the way it looks after its members is reflected in society at large. The elderly and the very young, the handicapped and the mentally ill are best cared for within the family, not in institutions. We cannot, of course, suddenly switch everyone from institutions to home without making the necessary vital adjustments to provide support for the family. This is especially important as, in society today, the family is going through rapid change and many individuals do not find themselves in a traditional family: they may be part of a one-parent family; grandparents with, in effect, no family; or members of a commune or some other social unit.

The family should have an impact on the local community. This may include networks of neighbours who regard it as a normal part of life,

Caring for each other. By giving a helping hand within the community, the young gain the wisdom of the old and the old gain security from the young.

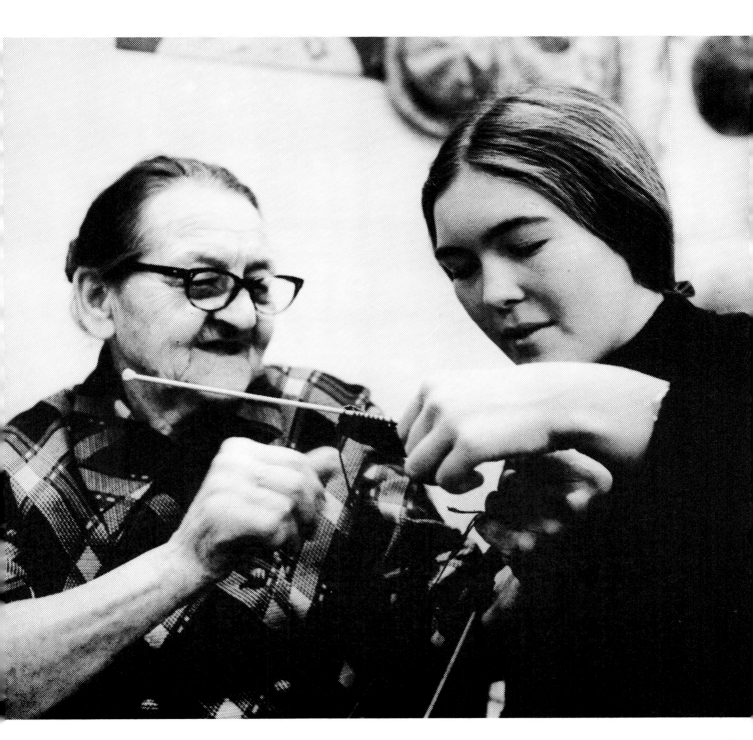

not charity, to assist independent older people with their shopping, give them lifts, or ensure that the local bus service also caters for the elderly.

Health also means the promotion of facilities such as sports centres. They are as vital a part of wellbeing as the medical centre. They should not be merely a sort of political gift, bestowed on a town 20 years after it has been built.

As well as the home and the community, there is the place of work, often the place which is most crucial to a person's health. While we spend much of our lives and energy at work, it is there that we are tempted to pay least attention to our health. Apart from dealing with obvious risks such as dangerous machinery, dangerous floor surfaces, or bad lighting, we need to ensure that we do not, for example, get bad backs, become overweight from sedentary occupations, develop worries that give us ulcers, or take up the habit of smoking to cope with the pressure.

The sports centre is not a luxury to be enjoyed only by affluent societies but a vital part of community services. It can help ensure a healthier and more productive population which wastes less money on trying to cure the diseases of the unfit

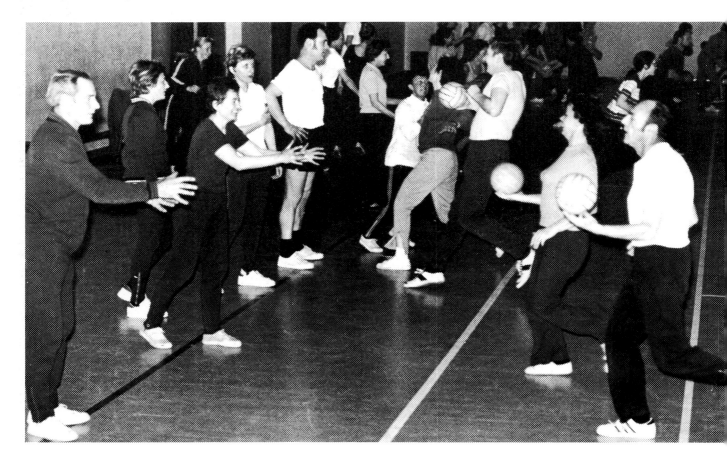

. . . who tend to over-eat and under-exercise, creating problems not only for themselves but also for society which must provide for cures when they collapse.

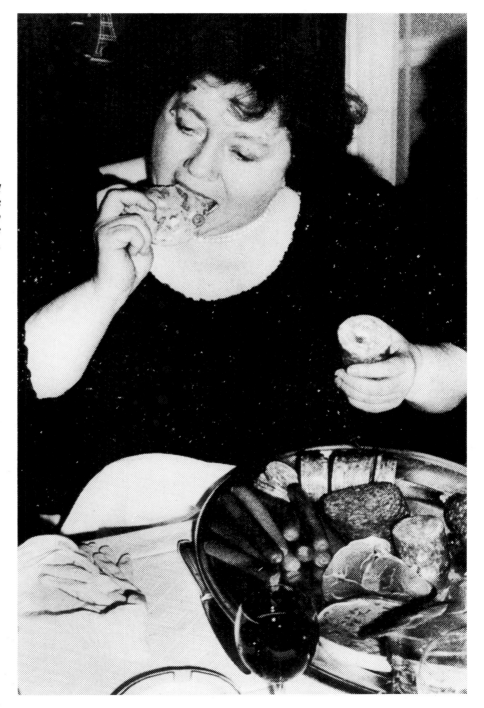

Sharing decisions

We need a fundamental shift in the way decisions are taken in the present health care systems to ensure that individuals and the wider groups they represent have a real role in determining their health. Decision-making in this field has been mainly in the hands of the medical profession and then usually only of those at the top end of the scale, not primary medical care personnel. If, as Dr Mahler says, health is to spring from within the community, those who have been responsible mainly for curing illnesses and not necessarily promoting health can no longer expect to maintain their monopoly of decision-making. What is required is not a straight shift of power from one group to another but rather a sharing of decision-making in the community. If there is to be common action, all should feel they are involved and have the ability to influence the outcome. Full involvement of the community in the new health strategy will mean a sharing of the decision-making process, at local, regional, and national level.

Consumer councils with power

Community participation is virtually non-existent in the primary care systems of most countries — the health facilities have developed as a service *to* the population rather than as a service *for* and *with* the population. A key suggestion in the Strategy is that there should be bodies such as national health councils or commissions of citizens, as both users and providers of the new community care. These would give grass-roots support and create public pressure to ensure that health for all is a realistic achievement for the turn of the century. Self-managing groups of users and providers of services already decide on all matters of health care in Yugoslavia, for example.

The involvement of the people does not mean that they can indulge in the narrow sectoral battles of the past, where health for all has too often meant high technology with all the drawbacks and no advantages. Participation would not only make the population more satisfied; it would also make the services more effective. In the commissions or councils people from all walks of life would be involved so that there is proper consultation before decisions are taken. The commissions would also act as watchdogs and support interest groups when desirable. At local level the support might be for a new pedestrian crossing for children near a school. At national level it could be a decision whether to permit construction of a new factory to help a depressed area. In both cases a local or national health council could ensure that financial or political aspects alone did not become the biggest deciding factor; that the local authority should not refuse a necessary crossing on budgetary grounds alone; or that the government should not offer massive tax concessions for the new factory and, at the same time, not provide money to ensure that social services were adequate. In both cases the health council would see that the health element was not sacrificed for short-term gains to the long-term detriment of health.

New political role for the people

This gives the people a new political role — not just a vote in parliamentary elections, but regular, direct involvement in the decision-making process. Too often the delegation of political power to representatives means the abandonment of responsibility by the individual citizen. This would be a great loss to real participation in devising a health strategy for the community. The community must act as a force for change in local and national government throughout every sector of public life. The exact nature of its future involvement in the field of health will depend on cultural and social factors. However, there should be a commitment to the increasing representation of the consumer on policy-forming and decision-making bodies so that he can take more responsibility in the organization of health services, from health promotion to hospital care.

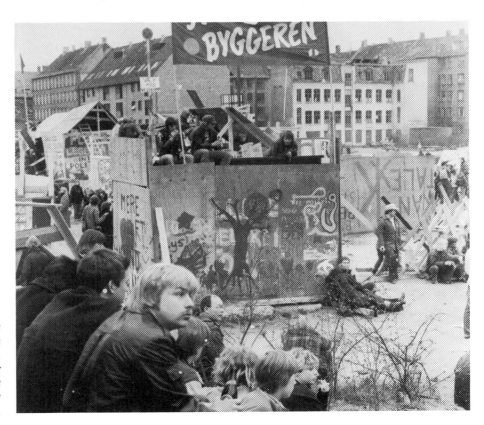

Power to the people. Protests arise at plans to build on much-needed open space. Involving people in health planning may not only avoid such protests but also ensure that their primary needs are known and provided for.

Power to women

Different governments and societies in the European Region will certainly have a variety of views on the composition of such commissions. In all countries, however, there is room for a very strong participation by women in them. It is essential that women are given the political role that is commensurate with their involvement in health in the community.

Any country that wishes to develop its human resources to meet the challenges of the twenty-first century must acknowledge that the health of a nation is a key factor for progress in any field, from education to industrialization. Women, as workers either in the home or outside, are vital to that factor. Yet there are glaring inequalities in the status of women, in terms not only of the rights and privileges available to them but also of their opportunity to determine how the rights and privileges of society are shared out. Women bear most of the burden of raising children and ensuring good nutrition and health in the family: the mother is never allowed to be sick — she is simply expected to cope. If health is to be part of every aspect of life, women have a right to make decisions in this area where they have always been expected to carry the greatest responsibility. It can justifiably be said that the European and Global Strategies for Attaining Health for All by the Year 2000 will fail unless the importance of the woman's role is recognized.

Such recognition will help change the current misinterpretation of responsibilities in child-rearing. It can be argued cogently that education and child-rearing have become overdependent on semi-professionals and professionals in matters that rarely need their skills and experience. It is women, not obstetricians, who should be encouraged to take decisions about pregnancy. It is they who should examine the use of sophisticated technology in maternity hospitals and obstetric wards. They should decide what is more appropriate for them and not tamely accept the obstetrician's decisions. The growth of women's organizations emphasizing and promoting self-care and self-reliance in health is nothing more than a reassertion of a natural role. Women in the community and family networks have been providing this supportive role for centuries in order to help meet their health needs.

Least of all should it be said that there is an inherent conflict among the various roles that women play as mothers, family members, and breadwinners. The fact that they are actually able to play these roles at the moment with so little support from society is an indication that they should not drop some of them. Rather, they should maintain them, if need be with the help of extra resources from the community purse.

As women take a more active role in work outside the home families must be given the support needed when they wish to have children. Self-care and community care must not mean putting more work on women.

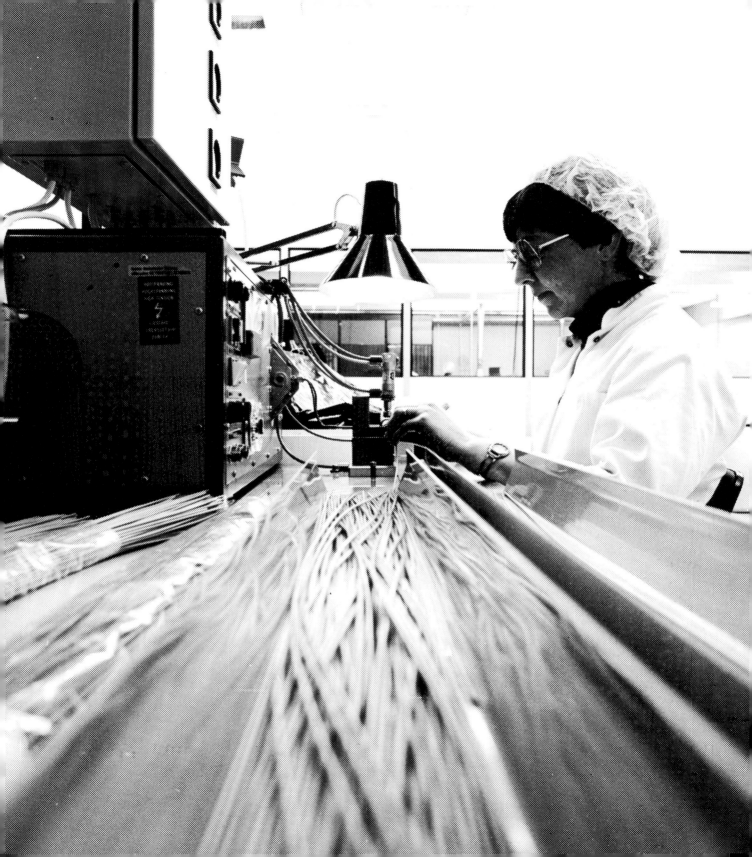

Self-management in health care

With the spread of the effects of the industrial revolution, life began to become more complex and specialized and the health care establishment became correspondingly more complex. In the developed countries of the world treatment in hospitals actually causes additional medical problems for many patients.

> Hospital-acquired infections are one of the main causes of morbidity and mortality in hospitalized patients at the present time, leading directly or indirectly to an enormous increase in the cost of hospital care and to the emergence of new health hazards for the community. Although some success has been achieved in controlling infections spreading in hospitals, recent advances in biomedical technology and therapeutics are producing greater numbers of highly susceptible patients, and this is aggravated by the occurrence of transferable resistance to antibiotics in pathogenic organisms. (2)

While we have examined the defects of hospitals, we have failed to monitor those most important components of self-care: family members caring for each other; help from relatives and friends; self-help by social groups among alcoholics, drug addicts, the handicapped, the blind, etc. We know, however, that at least two thirds of all illness is cared for without professional intervention. For the one third of patients who seek professional help, 75% have already practised some type of self-care before going to the doctor. Doctors themselves have reckoned that this preliminary self-care is effective in 90% of cases. These findings are particularly significant since they come from countries where professional care is free of charge and universally available.

Thirty years ago the medical profession provided diabetics with needles and syringes so that they could give themselves their own injections. Diabetics needed an injection and a urine test every day, could not be kept in hospital for the purpose, and could not be visited every day. Not only do the patients now look after their injections perfectly well; the doctor also has more time to exercise better supervision and offer his skills to a larger number of people.

Women do it better

We have already said that women should exercise a much greater role in the shift by society towards a new health strategy. It is worth examining their role in some detail because it has much to teach both lay people and health professionals on how to move away from curative and towards preventive medicine.

Self-care or self-management is sometimes dismissed out of hand as being useless. The facts clearly say otherwise. Returning specifically to the role of women, we can see an even more important change that

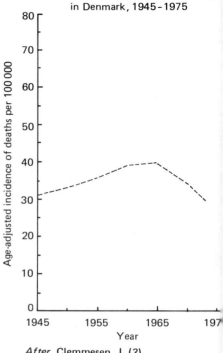

Mortality rate from cervical cancer, in Denmark, 1945-1975

Age-adjusted incidence of deaths per 100 000

Year

After Clemmesen, J. (*3*).

Self-care begins at home. Beginning in 1962, home kits for detecting cervical cancer were mailed to women in Copenhagen who took their own samples and sent them to the laboratory. The response was so positive, and so many cases were detected at an early, curable stage, that by 1965 mortality from cervical cancer had begun to decrease. The trauma of going to a physician had been removed, with positive results.

Bringing health care to the people. Primary health care services no longer wait for sick people to come to a clinic, often too late, but involve health promotion through regular visits to people in their home

60

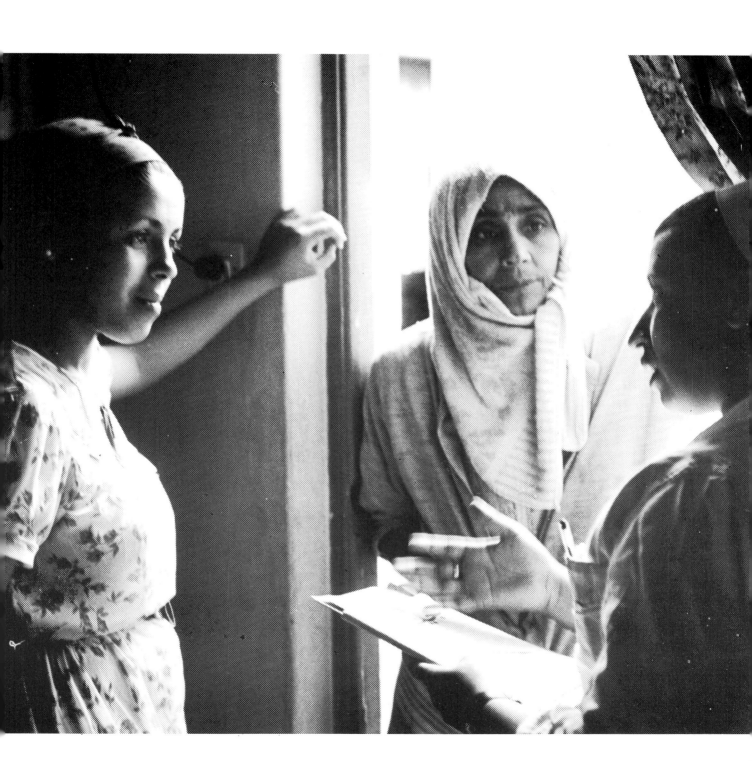

has taken place in the last few years. Whereas the doctors gave the diabetics their equipment, women's self-help groups have actually taken equipment from the doctors. To some extent this active move by women grew out of their often poor relationship with the male-dominated medical profession. There are a number of conditions that cause women discomfort, pain and embarrassment but to which doctors have paid relatively little attention. These are easily detected and treated, and self-help groups now use the vaginal speculum for the purpose, as well as to examine for signs of cancer or other conditions. It has begun to allow women to take their bodies back from the medical profession. By regular examination they begin to know when they are healthy, or when they need attention. The same principle is applied in breast examination for cancer, which all women can and should practise.

"Demedicalization"

The demedicalization of health will certainly release the doctor to do a better job for us, but it must come from the community as well as the profession. The caring relationship mentioned earlier has largely disappeared from the health services. It is not just the necessarily aseptic walls of the hospital we are talking about. It is the fact that death very rarely occurs in the home now as something natural — instead the patient is taken away to die. Thus, families find it more difficult to cope with sudden loss because death has been hidden from them. Similarly, too many babies are born in hospital. The means exist today for most of us to have our children born at home in complete safety. We need to find a balance between making home more like hospital in terms of good medical attention, and hospital more like home in terms of familiarity and comfort.

Public debate

These are some of the changes that women's groups are pressing for in growing numbers throughout the world. The reorganization of the national health services that will be needed will require local, regional and national debate by every group in society including trade unions, professional bodies, and voluntary bodies of all kinds. There is also an international context that goes beyond the European Region. Groups involved with world development and the Third World will want to ensure that the Regional Strategy forms part of the Global Strategy, which WHO is pursuing within the framework of the United Nations and through its coordinating role.

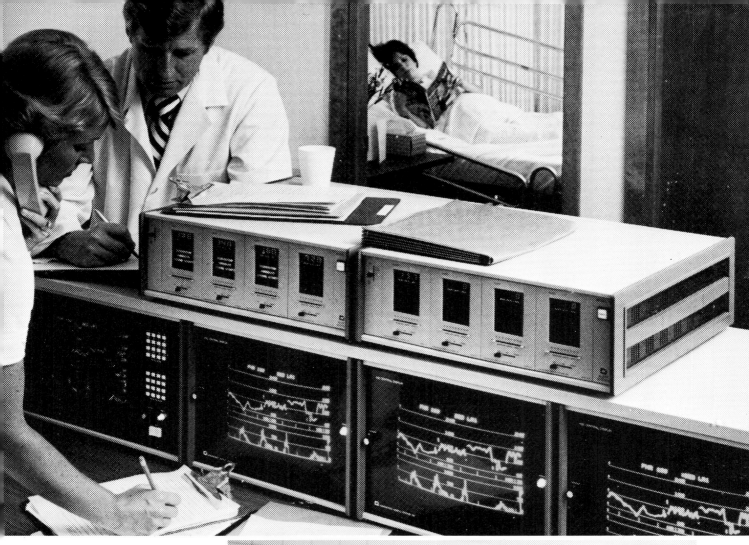

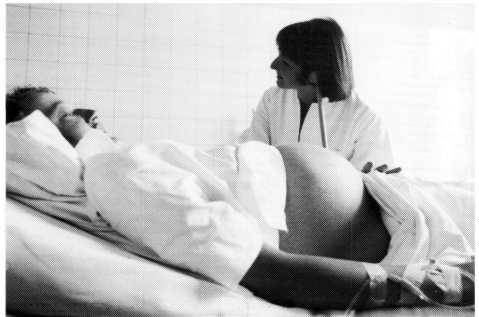

Foetal monitoring old and new: machine versus midwife. The over-medicalization of many natural processes has meant that high-technology machines have become a barrier to the human contact which can be so valuable in health care. Such a barrier may more than offset the higher efficiency expected from machines such as this multiple foetal monitor.

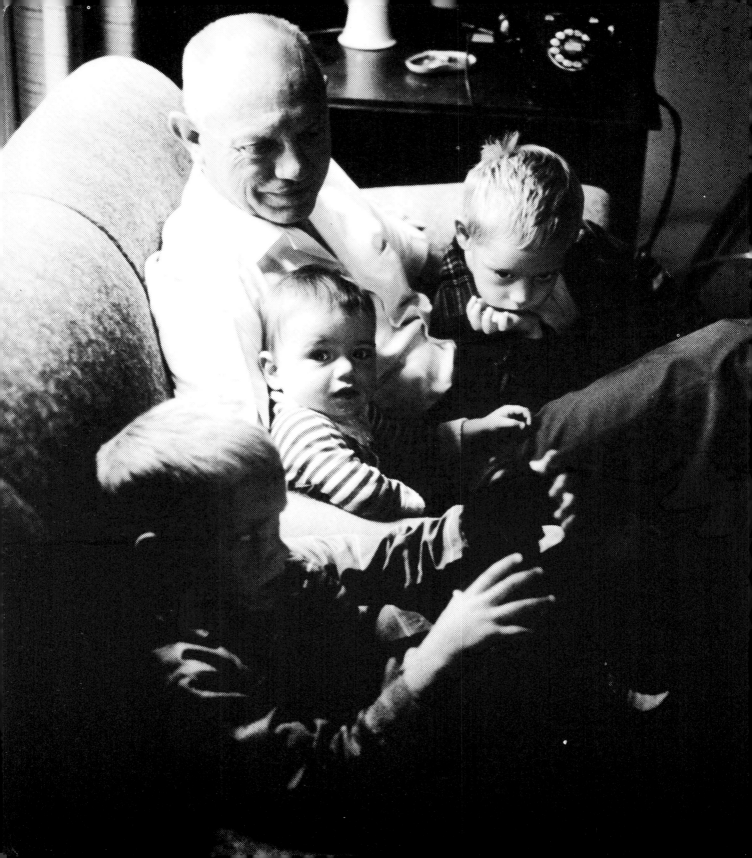

5.

New challenge
for the health profession

Medical schools and reform

It is reasonably fair to assume that the health profession will wish to play a leading role in the direction society must take to achieve the new health strategy. This is not to say that it will be an easy task. It is the very advances in research and medical education that prompted Dr Mahler recently to pose the following questions.

— Do graduates think and behave in terms of "health" rather than of "disease"? That is to say, do they apply techniques of prevention and health promotion and not only those of cure and rehabilitation?

— Do graduates think and behave in terms of the family and community rather than in terms of the individual sick patient?

— Do graduates think and behave in terms of membership of a health team consisting of doctors, nurses, and other health workers, as well as social scientists?

— Do graduates think and behave in terms of making the best and most effective use of the financial and material resources available?

— Do graduates think and behave in terms of their country's patterns of health and disease and its relevant priorities?

If the answer to all these questions is in the affirmative, then the medical school is going some considerable way to preparing a graduate whose training is relevant to the health needs of modern society. If, however, some of the answers are not an unequivocal "yes", there is urgent need to re-examine the whole philosophy and programme of the school concerned. (1)

Serving the community

The medical profession must look closely at what serving the health needs of the community means. If community care is to develop from within the community the doctor can become a catalyst in a new team of people caring for health, ranging from the active consumer to the expert members of a health team including people such as the midwife and the social worker. Any good community care philosophy will ensure that the right approach to health by the individual through self-care fits harmoniously into a speedy referral system if the individual develops a health condition needing more than self-care. This will mean that the right technology will be available to the right person at the right time. By ensuring that specialization plays its correct role, not one distorted by misguided public demand, the specialist will be able to offer a valid service.

Who does what and when?

Human resources will play a fundamental role in the achievement of health for all by the year 2000. Apart from the involvement of citizens, new types of staff will need to be trained. Governments will have to take vigorous but carefully planned action to provide enough health personnel of the appropriate types to implement their strategies. The aim must not be quantity but quality, the right people for the right job, with completely new attitudes. There are already parts of Europe where there are too many physicians, yet nobody enjoys any better health for that. Good planning will avoid wasteful overproduction of health personnel, a point worth remembering since most of the physicians who will be active by the end of the century are studying now or have already completed their studies. It also means that today's health workers will need new attitudes, not only towards their work in the community but also towards the role of the nonprofessional.

Health personnel in the future will work together more in teams. Thus, the way nurses, doctors, radiologists, etc., are all separately trained will have to be re-examined. If they are to see patients as persons rather than as cases in their particular specialty, they can gain a great deal from each other by training together. This applies not only to knowledge but also to working relationships, particularly for the doctor who has often in the past tended to be the overlord, "assisted" by others. There have been disturbing cases where new primary care training systems have tried to put nurses and doctors on an equal level and nurses have assumed the dominating attitudes of the doctors to those nursing colleagues who were not on the course. If members of the health team are to work together on the basis of what they can offer, rather than on what their rank is, the new attitude must start at medical school.

The other important requirement is that medical graduates should have regular refresher courses throughout their careers. The overworked general practitioners in the past had no such provision so, to their patients' detriment, they were not able to continue developing their skills. This applies equally to other primary health care workers and nurses. The postgraduate centres that have been established throughout the United Kingdom for use by general practitioners are an example of a trend that should be widely followed.

Evaluation and cooperation
The changes needed must be the object of adequate and imaginative research, especially in the design of the primary health care programmes and of new training courses that are community-oriented and integrated with the local health services. They should not just be based on a hospital, and the main emphasis should be on prevention, primary care, and long-term care. The effects of these changes should be monitored constantly and in close consultation with community representatives and

the professions. Consultation must include the vital nonprofessional workers such as volunteer hospital visitors, the Samaritans, and self-help groups among the disabled.

Such new training and monitoring offers an excellent opportunity for cooperation between colleges and research centres on a regional basis. The Strategy suggests that a network of regional training centres can be developed leading to valuable cooperation among national education systems. Much can be gained by increasing cooperation with the Third World, through exchanges of people and results in both directions, and of facilities to train specialists and teachers. In this way some countries can avoid the wasteful mistakes that others have already made.

The "family nurse" knows her clients, visiting them not only in sickness but also in health. Aware of family problems before they become serious, she can call in other members of the primary care team when needed.

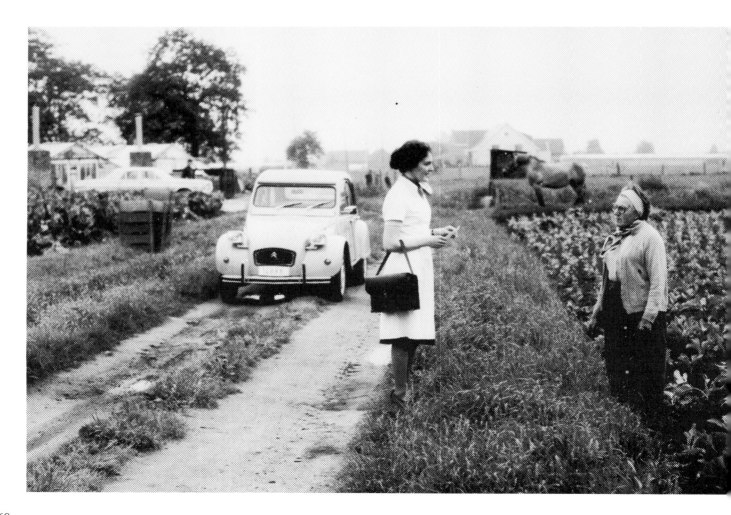

PRIMARY CARE TEAMS

Within the total philosophy of community care it will be necessary to develop a satisfactory primary care team, through research, consultation with the consumer, and trial and error. Some forms of primary health care already exist in various parts of the Region. However, there has been no adequate research into the general role of such care. There are fortunately exceptions of some value such as pilot studies in Finland where considerable progress has been made (2). Such research is an essential part of the Strategy, but it is already possible to see some of the forms this primary care could take in, for example, nursing services, new health centres, and consumer cooperation.

Nursing

The organization of public health and community nursing varies widely among the countries of the Region. In some, nurses are integral parts of primary health care teams; in others, they work in almost total isolation. Elsewhere, community nurses are independent practitioners paid on a fee-for-service basis. There are often no definite links with domestic help or social work services. The vast majority of nurses work in hospitals and there is no practicable way at the moment of providing appropriate care outside the hospital, even though it would cost less and be preferred by patients and their families. In the new scheme of things they would have a great deal to offer. After a mother or other relative, it is usually the nurse who is the closest monitor of a person's health. Whether in the hospital, the home, the office, or the factory, nurses rank high in contact with the consumer and are of vital importance to any team.

At present public health nurses or health visitors often have far too many families to visit; they can do little more than call on those with known medical or perhaps social problems, change a dressing here, or follow up on a difficult pregnancy there. If they were responsible for a smaller population they could visit *all* the families regularly and become a kind of "family nurse", with an even better personal relationship with those they help than the former family doctors had. They would then be in a position to be aware of lifestyle problems – a teenager under examination stress, a mother beginning to drink too much, a father threatened with redundancy – and help the families guard against the associated threats to health. They could call in a social worker or refer patients who need a doctor's skills only when necessary, so saving the doctor's valuable time. The savings in terms of ill health prevented and productivity gained would soon more than repay their cost in the primary care team.

Under fee-for-service payment systems people pay for specific medical services, but even if a practitioner is paid for a regular check-up or for advice to someone on how to change his lifestyle, the service is poorly rewarded. Where doctors are paid according to the number of patients on their list, curative services must be provided but the system may not require them to provide counselling and check-ups. For these and other reasons (not the least of which is the way medical students are taught), the most important personal preventive services are grossly underprovided for.

The implication of the growing opinion that primary care must be strengthened and the hospital relieved of demands that are better and possibly more economically satisfied elsewhere is that primary health care can no longer be adequately provided by single-handed medical practitioners. They need supporting staff and coordination of the staff needs some kind of organization, not for its own sake but so as to be able to respond better to consumer needs (3).

Nevertheless, the individual health practitioner is still not uncommon in many European countries, and his position is quite often reinforced by the way national health system payments are organized. Some would like to see the pattern change in favour of group practice. However, the specific rights of the individual medical practitioner continue to be important in group practice and may perhaps be a brake on the development of broader attitudes towards primary health care. In spite of this, the major trend at present is probably towards health centres or polyclinics. Curative and preventive care is available in both, although neither has yet achieved its full potential.

A new kind of centre?

Health centres as described above are based on a traditional health service system. We are, however, at the threshold of a whole new approach as, for example, when the social welfare and health services of a community are collected together in one place. By covering all aspects of life, they could really then be called *health* centres. There the local population could bring problems about its children, the elderly, working adults, or unemployed young persons. It would be the place to which people naturally turned whatever the requirement — health promotion, prevention, first aid, or primary diagnosis — and would perhaps find encouragement to try to solve the problems within the family or at the place of work. This sort of service could provide better care for the individual in the community than the existing, often fragmented, health and welfare services. At such a centre the individual could meet a person who acted in his interest. It need not necessarily be a physician — it might be a psychologist, occupational therapist, employ-

The "family doctor" provides personal service. While growth health centres and polyclini helps the development of broad attitudes toward primary heal care, personal preventive servic are still grossly underprovide

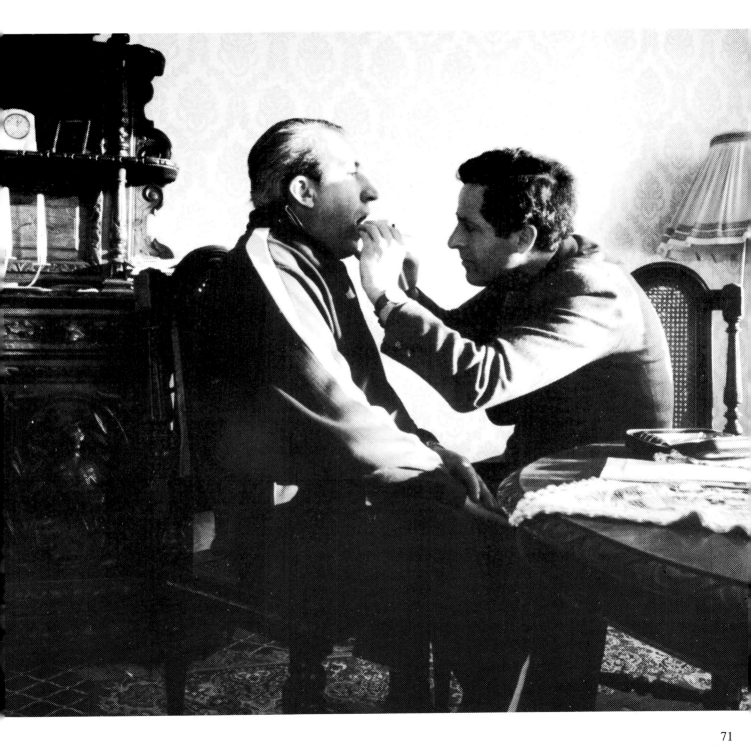

ment counsellor, public health nurse, or midwife. Where an individual had several problems there would be a much better chance of finding solutions if those with the ability to help were working together, for the individual's problems do not stay in separate compartments — they all have a combined effect (3).

More teamwork with the consumer

The basic conclusion is that community care, from self-help to sophisticated services, requires far more teamwork than in the past. This means that other health workers no longer just assist the doctor in treating a passive patient. The patients themselves need to be active, participating consumers availing themselves of the services they consider should be supplied by a health team. The mystique enveloping medicine is disappearing for the average educated person. The attitude of uncritical acceptance of everything the doctor says and does will not suffice for the years ahead. The caring role of nonprofessional personnel is increasingly being recognized in the European Region, although we are still only at the beginning of this trend.

Danger of complacency

A word of warning is appropriate at this stage. Because there is a wealth of medical skill available at the moment, physicians and public may both say: "We are well served, thank you. We have enough doctors". A large number of doctors, however, would prefer to see a more comprehensive approach taken towards health, and of course they will need the willing support and leadership of those who actually run the present system.

Expansion of traditional roles

The medical schools have a leading role to play in helping change direction and break down some of the artificial barriers within the essentially hierarchical health profession. The change in approach will, it is hoped, increase the professional incentive to study the problems that lie ahead in relation to the mentally ill, the handicapped, the old, rural populations, migrant workers, and the unemployed. These are the new fields of professional excellence for the up-and-coming young doctor, research worker, and community health worker. Society may have to look again at how people are rewarded for work in these fields. They must no longer be regarded as the dead end of the profession. Health professionals have before them a dramatic new role in addition to the exercise of their clinical skills: that of health leaders, educators, guides, and generators, of simpler and more socially acceptable technologies. To fulfil this role they will require a combination of sagacity, scientific and technical knowledge, social understanding, managerial acumen and, above all, political persuasiveness.

Is high technology always appropriate? Most children could be born at home in complete safety, but if babies have to be born in hospital, women should be given more say in the use of sophisticated equipment in maternity wards.

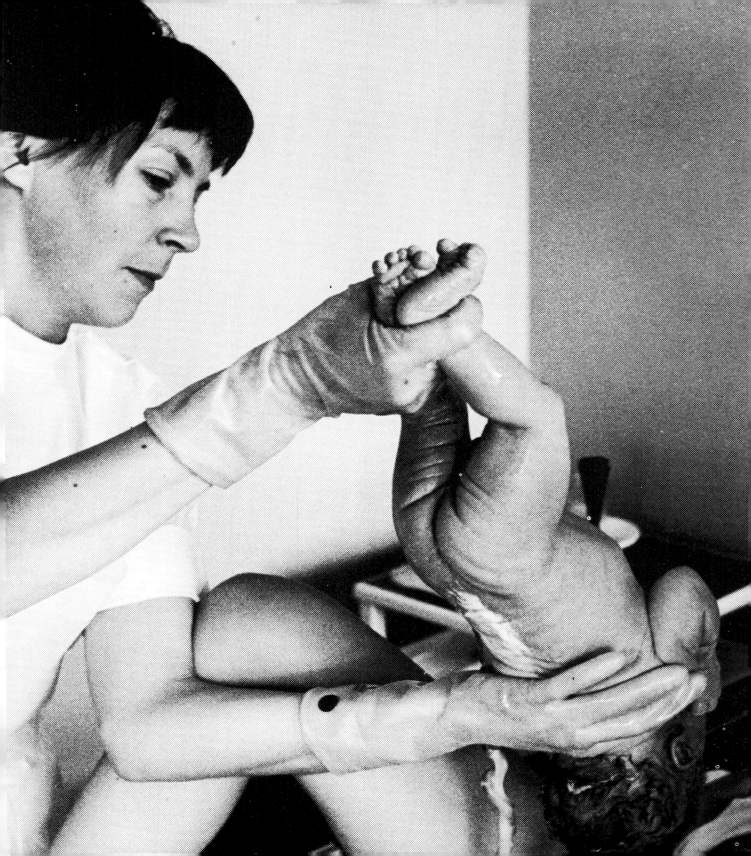

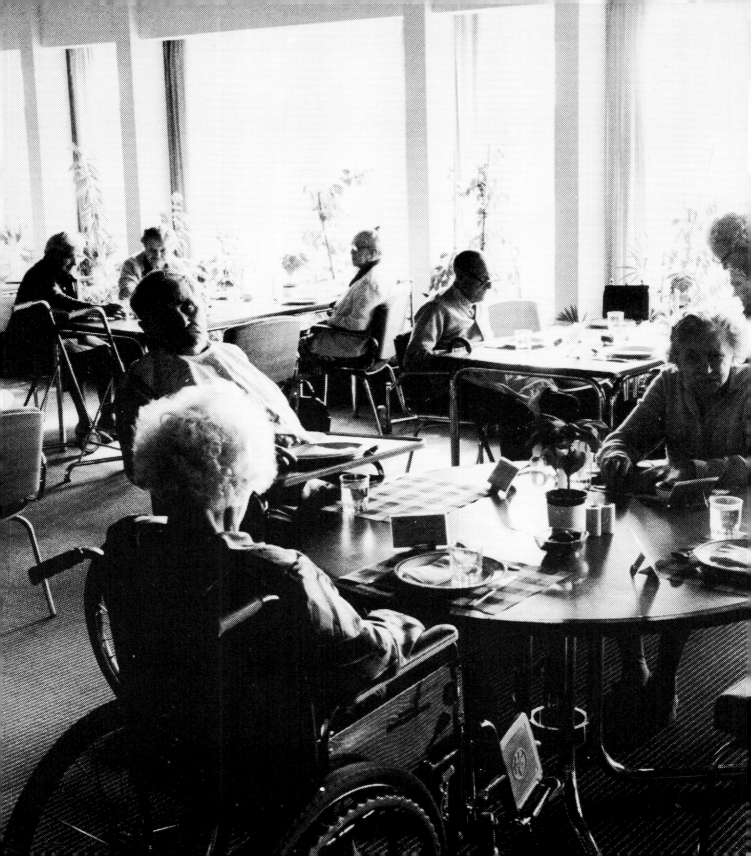

6.

New health for all

This chapter considers the needs of various groups in society, using the elderly as an example. In the rest of the book we shall try to avoid dealing with people in isolated groups and instead refer to the themes of the Strategy to bring health to whole communities, or at least to individuals as part of communities.

The three central themes of the Strategy are health as a way of life; the battle to prevent disease; and community care that is accessible, adequate, and acceptable to all. All these elements must constantly run through the various stages of life.

TARGET GROUPS AND THE ELDERLY

Most countries of the Region have low birth rates and these are unlikely to change, so the population will probably remain much the same. However, there are going to be more and more elderly people with the chronic diseases of old age and improved services will be needed to postpone their mental and physical decline (1). The expected success of preventive programmes will add to those needs, and the trend towards moving house on retirement is likely to place increasing strain on the health services of the areas selected for retirement. Support will have to be provided for elderly people within their own homes and in their own communities.

The special needs of the elderly show how they fit, as a target group, into the interdependent community as a whole. They are not a problem any more than are the handicapped, single mothers, the mentally ill, or migrant workers, as long as the needs of such groups are recognized as something the community will always have to respond to and make regular provision for. In most instances the way to meet those needs will be self-evident and can be selected from the suggestions in the Strategy summarized under the three headings: lifestyles, prevention, and care.

Some perspective can be given to the idea of target groups by consideration of the disabled. The year 1981 was the year of the disabled who, out of a world population of over four thousand million people, account for more than 10%. They are not a minor group — they form a significant proportion of the population, whether their disabilities are caused by genetic defects, birth trauma, accidents at home, on the road or at work, malnutrition, alcohol, drugs, or industrial diseases.

These groups already do a great deal to care for themselves. In Norway parents with haemophiliac children have banded together to define the limitations of their children's activities and provide themselves the treat-

Aging Europe. One of the most important groups in society is the elderly, both in numbers and in special needs. By the year 2000 they will make up about a fifth of most European countries' populations, including a growing number of over 80-year-olds. The community must play its part in providing them with accessible and adequate care to prevent their premature mental and physical decline.

Population trends in the European Region: estimated percentage of population aged 60 years and over

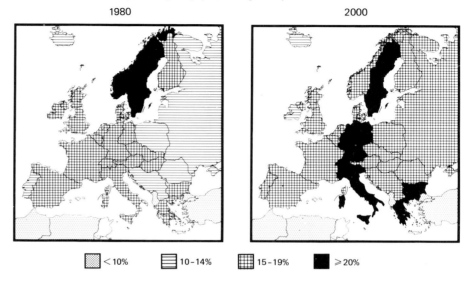

1980   2000

☒ < 10%   ☰ 10 - 14%   ▦ 15 - 19%   ■ ≥ 20%

Population trends in the European Region: estimated percentage of population aged 80 years and over

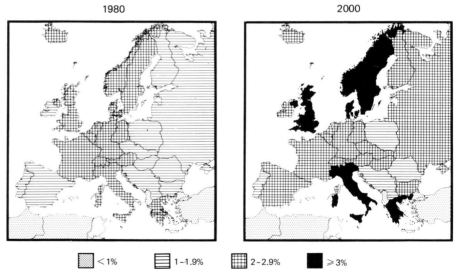

1980   2000

☒ < 1%   ☰ 1 - 1.9%   ▦ 2 - 2.9%   ■ ≥ 3%

Source: United Nations (*2*).

ment and care necessary to manage this chronic condition. In so doing, they and their children have begun to learn to accept and enjoy life within those limitations. Through self-support, they have eliminated some of the severe psychological effects — as they could probably never have done in a purely hospital-based caring system. As a result, in contrast with the increasing trend towards more hospitalization for all other groups of illnesses, increased hospital care has not been needed for this group.

Each country or community must obviously work out its own plans for tackling its needs within the broad framework of the Strategy for Attaining Health for All by the Year 2000. We might all seriously begin to think, however, of ways in which "normal" people ought to start changing. Why are signs in public places big enough only for normal people to read, when 10% have marked visual impairment and many more would have difficulty in picking out such signs. Similarly, for the hard-of-hearing, why not add a text to the screen in news and other programmes to make it easier for them to watch television?

The preventive and curative needs of the group aged 65 years and over are summarized in the Strategy document as follows:

The needs of the elderly

Cardiovascular diseases, cancer, mental disorders, rheumatisms, arthritis and permanent disability are the major health problems among the elderly. These are often difficult to distinguish from the general problems of aging. To all this is added physical, economic and social difficulties that together create a situation of dependence and disorientation. In the case of the dying, there are problems of providing emotional support and preventing isolation, and the excessive use of high technology can lead to the unnecessary prolongation of suffering.

The elderly have a vital social role to play. They are usually the most experienced members of society. They may have more physical needs than the rest of the family, but quite often they are the least demanding. If allowed, they can play a positive role in the rearing of children, providing stability in the home and offering parents a chance of relaxation from the demands of their children. They can, because of their past experience, provide a psychological anchor in times of stress.

It is wrong to consider the elderly as a burden. This is the view of a society that has come to see the institutionalization of old people as part of the cheese-paring that seems to dominate our supermarket lives. Society could reassess the role of the elderly, provide them with houses and flats in which they could manage for themselves, and make home help services more easily available when necessary. Alternatively, houses for parents with young families could also have accommodation for grandparents who could help in the house. In this fashion we might begin to appreciate the value of the older person again.

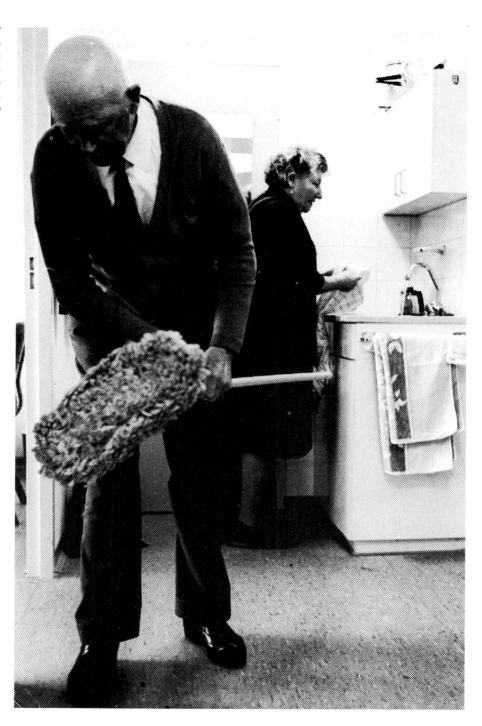

Staying at home. Many elderly people who are now confined to old people's homes or even hospitals could be living happily (and much less expensively) at home if a little more effort were made to meet their special housing needs.

While the elderly can offer much to the community, it should be accepted that they do require planned help from other social groups. They are a good indicator of how far we have moved towards a really caring community, not just because we look after them better but because we shall have shown how we have given old people an active role in life and not left them in a dead end with nothing to look forward to except a gradual decline in standard of living, growing isolation, and perhaps a lonely death from hypothermia.

We also need to look very closely at compulsory retirement at a fixed age. Tragically, in many cases this means the end of a life bound up with work and then, literally, death shortly afterwards. In a climate of increased productivity and lower manning levels, the solution accepted by unions and management is often natural wastage, a phrase that is uncomfortably near the truth. Many people are more than able to keep on working after the retiring age, and need to keep on working because for them this is part of a healthy lifestyle. For them, retirement is accompanied by the same stresses as dismissal or redundancy. They may not be able to work at the same level as before, but there is little justification for making room for young people by creating a health hazard for the old and often, in effect, killing them off. Far more attention needs to be given to finding the best ways of ensuring that the transition from work to retirement does not lead to the "pension disease" or to the grave.

Care for the elderly
We should be able to devise a system to ensure that, if the elderly are living at home and need hospital care, it should be for the minimum time. Any reorganization of a national health system should see that people spend as little time in hospital as possible and instead get better care from the community care structure at home or at the local level. Why should this not apply to the elderly? Day care and day assessment facilities for them would remove much of the anxiety they suffer when faced with hospitalization. Many tests probably need to be done in hospital only because no one has bothered to make the equipment easily available locally or because the doctor or specialist finds it more convenient to have the patient in hospital. Old people are often prone to confusion and anxiety, and a home-based approach would help reduce these. If we cannot prevent all the diseases of old age we can concentrate on the prevention of unnecessary suffering.

Now that there is going to be a larger elderly population in the world by the turn of the century than ever before, we have much to learn from those countries in the south of the European Region that have retained many of the best features of the extended family and involve the elderly in the ordinary life of the family and community.

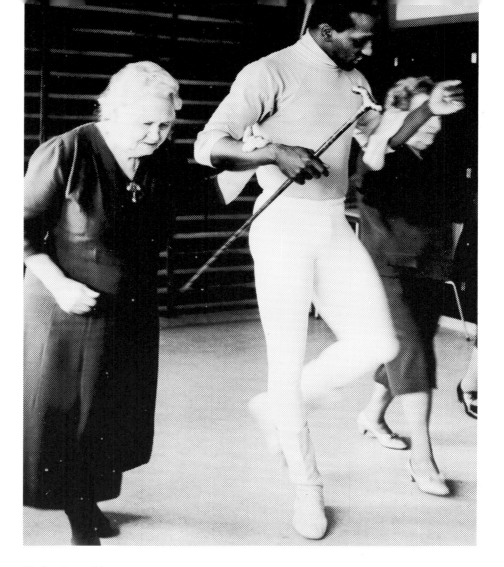

Enjoying old age

A change in national policy should take proper account of the implications of meeting the needs of a much larger number of older people. Better coordination between social and health services will both improve the services and save money. More research into new technology for the elderly could help them make the best of their health.

We must remove the stigma that has now been attached to the elderly and stop their growing devaluation in the eyes of society. Those working with the elderly are wrongly regarded as having a low status by the medical profession and often by the public too. Caring requires at least as much skill and knowledge as prevention or curing. On a par with the massive investment in the search for spectacular drugs, there should be research to understand the basic processes of aging, the aim being not simply to add years to life but to add life to years.

Society should welcome the growing number of old people we have with us with warmth and pride. Not only do parents and children live longer in each other's company, but extended old age is also a great tribute to the advances that society has made in recent years in conquering many of the killing diseases of previous centuries. Having spent so much time and effort in ensuring that people live to a ripe old age, it seems foolish for society to throw the benefits away — nor must society forget that all of us will, in due course, join the ranks of the elderly.

NEEDS AT OTHER AGES

The emphasis on lifestyle, prevention, and care touched on above for the elderly applies equally well, though in different ways, to other groups such as infants, children, expectant mothers, the handicapped, the

Defying the law . . .
. . . or defying death.
Accidents are the biggest
killer of young people. The
risk of death per mile travelled
on a motorcycle is 20 times
that in a car.

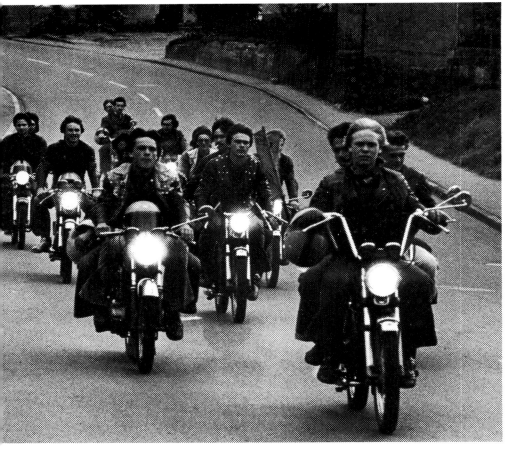

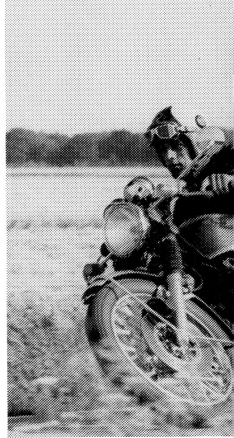

mentally ill, and the visually impaired. It would be wrong to maintain the traditional medical approach of separating these groups from the community — they are part and parcel of the community. The medical concept of high-risk groups has its uses, but it has its dangers, too, if carried too far.

A look at the preventive and curative needs of other age groups in society will help fit them into an overall plan where they are linked to each other in a natural framework. These are spelt out, from the original Strategy document, in the paragraphs below.

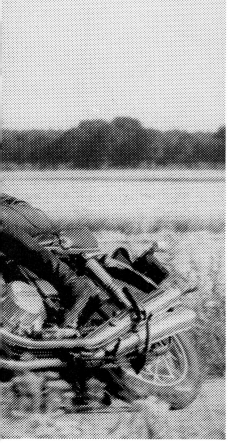

Join the professionals. Protective clothing helps prevent severe injuries. The use of a helmet reduces the risk of death in an accident by 40%.

Infants up to the age of one year

In the less developed parts of the Region infant mortality is almost 100 per 1000 live births owing to poverty, low standards of hygiene, poor nutrition and limited access to appropriate health care. In the industrialized countries the infant mortality rate continued to fall in the sixties and seventies, and by 1976 in the majority of countries it ranged between 10 and 30 per 1000 live births. There are, however, marked variations in mortality and morbidity among infants and young children, both among and within the wealthier countries. The main problems are the incidence of low birth weight and of congenital defects, some of which can be detected before birth. Perhaps because of the many complex factors in the environment of an industrial society which we do not really understand, and the fact that we are able to save people who would otherwise have died from congenital malformations, there may be an increase in those problems.

Children 1-14

This group also is prone to catching infectious diseases. In the less developed parts of the Region poor standards of nutrition and hygiene still create important problems, especially for children. All over the Region, accidents are a major cause of death and disability. This period is critical for the determination of values and lifestyles and the acquisition of undesirable habits, such as the abuse of alcohol, other drugs and tobacco. With the lowering of the age of puberty, the problem of early and unwanted pregnancy starts in this age group.

Adolescents and young adults 15-24

This group is characterized by unwanted pregnancies, sickness and death connected with childbearing, the "epidemic" of road traffic accidents, other accidents, suicide, alcohol and other drug misuse, and sexually transmitted diseases. Difficulties in identifying with the social environment, stress among school drop-outs and the unemployment of young people may be increasing their problems in fitting in with society around them, and so they develop disruptive lifestyles as a reaction to stress.

Adults 25-64

Road traffic and work accidents, mental diseases, cancer, heart disease, stroke and permanent disability are the major health problems with which this group must contend. Behind these lie such disruptive aspects of lifestyle as the abuse of alcohol, changes in family role, instability in employment, unemployment, and other social problems.

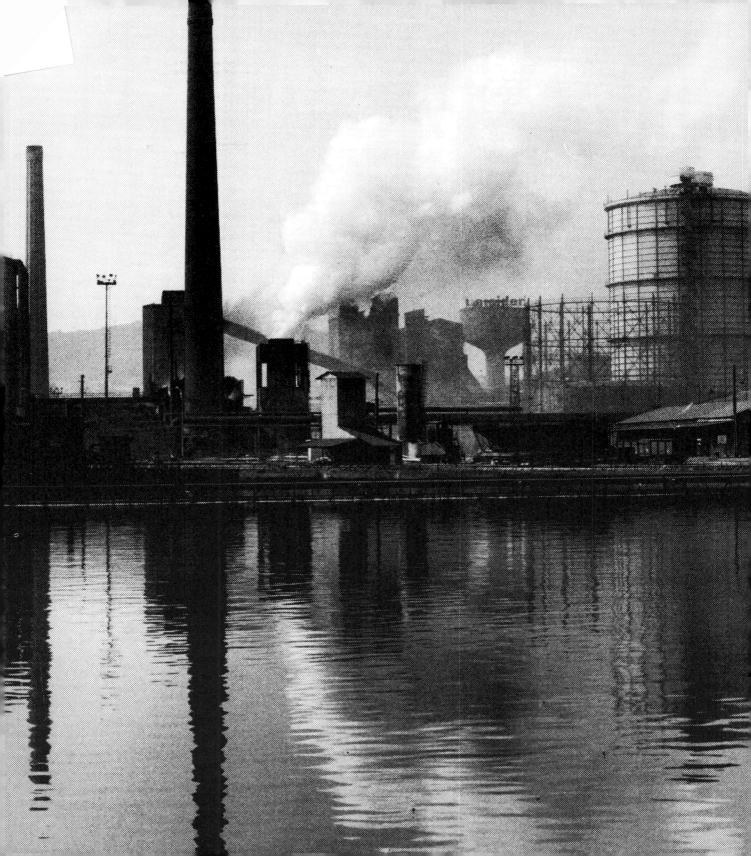

7.

Health as a way of life

As will be clear from what has gone before, the Strategy gives fresh emphasis to the theme of promoting new, healthy lifestyles as a way of life. By its very nature, this theme recurs constantly in this discussion. Detailed proposals will therefore not be spelled out again — only the basic principles will be outlined and points for action summarized.

Health consciousness

Since time immemorial politicians and philosophers have talked of the importance of raising the political consciousness of the masses. The time has now come to talk of raising their health consciousness. The greatest benefit will be to the individual — the one who suffers most when ill.

Pollution — pay now, save later

Health consciousness takes in wider horizons than individual health. Thus, most people now accept that the environment should not be polluted because of the danger to health. Some people, however, are not prepared to pay the cost, or else no one has worked out a suitable way of getting rid of a particular pollutant. Legislation is therefore needed to control, for example, the movement of dangerous products or the dumping of harmful wastes. Environmental control costs money, but it costs much more if control is not incorporated in the industrial or other plan. The traditional answer from industry is that it will put in the controls but, regretfully, must pass the cost on to the consumer. When the cost of control is high, however, and in times of economic recession even seems to threaten jobs, the temptation is to oppose control. This ignores the usually unseen health dangers that emerge only in the long term, as they did with asbestos. There are sound reasons for combating an approach that advocates the relaxation or non-imposition of control, whatever the reason advanced.

There are, indeed, many cases on record where industry has complained about the cost of cleaning up the environment and when it did so found it had a profitable by-product to sell. One instance is fluoride from brick kilns. Brick kilns produce highly dangerous amounts of fluoride, which in the past were found to be poisoning cows in neighbouring fields. The brick companies trapped the emissions and began selling the fluoride for safe, controlled use.

Although the worker may feel that his job will be affected, in fact jobs are often created by environmental controls, as experience in California has shown. The politician needs to consider subsidies to industry to help it install effective controls.

Escape to the open air or escape to hospital. Access to open space for exercise and recreation can mean the difference between health and hospitalization for millions who are daily subjected to the stress of city living

Selling health promotion

Health is so important and so beneficial to a nation that it ought to be promoted as something positive. Cigarette health warnings and posters showing the effects of alcoholism are negative in their impact; we need a positive approach to health in our environment, as something far more worthwhile acquiring than the coconut-palmed island where the natives live in the sun on martinis, nuts, and nothing else.

Health should be on our doorstep in the form of city parks for the urban dweller and nature and wildlife reserves all can use. Unfortunately, although the planners and politicians talk about the importance of these aspects of our life, they are the very first things to come under the economy axe. Yet they are as vital to our lungs as are the trees that make our cities breathe by recirculating oxygen and purifying the air.

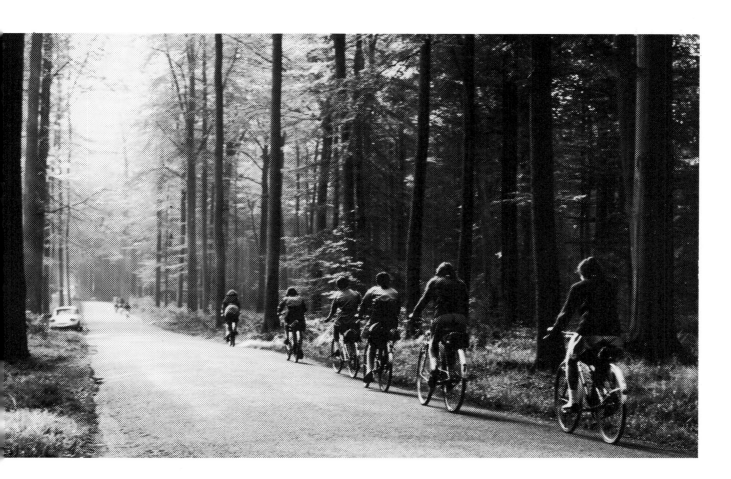

As community care networks form, they will offer a vehicle for the promotion of health in the home by parental example, as well as by contact with friends and neighbours and in the school. Anti-smoking campaigns in schools and on children's television are turning children into teachers of their parents. The office, the shopfloor, and the supermarket are also social networks where the message has to be spread. Health posters in factories and trade union offices must deal with more than just safety at work. We have the technology to make the home, too, a safe and healthy place if consumers and manufacturers put their minds to it.

A choice of lifestyles
It is in our choice of lifestyles that we can most affect the way we enjoy health as a way of life. It is a topsy-turvy world in which beautiful women and handsome men are used to advertise alcohol and cigarettes — two of the biggest causes of illness, accidents, and death in this century. Whatever legislation is enacted to prevent such advertising, there also needs to be a campaign, from the cradle onwards, to proclaim that it is the way of life without the cigarette and the bottle that enables people to enjoy life as well as to enjoy it for longer. We, as individuals, have the option of deciding for ourselves, but we must take steps to influence those who would influence us. Manufacturers and retailers have the greatest responsibility, but when children and parents are constantly bombarded with the wrong message, usually seductively put across, where does the blame really lie? There are many vested interests, from the worker and factory owner who earn a living producing the goods to the governments that make money directly or indirectly through taxes, that are unwilling to change the message. The whole community needs to discuss the problem and seek a solution, which may involve providing alternative ways of making a living for producers and traders, if necessary with subsidies.

The importance of sex
Part of the Strategy is to seek a greater understanding of the role that sexuality plays as one of the most powerful forces in society and in the life of an individual. The study of sex is not simply the study of human reproduction. It is also the study of its full psychological and social implications for all ages and all groups of society. We must move from the study of sexually transmitted diseases into research on how human sexuality fits into our overall development.

In 1960, only 3 medical schools out of 114 in the United States had formal training in the study of sex education. The progress was dramatic up to 1974, by which time 106 schools had instituted courses. A survey in 1975 found, however, that although 81% of 118 medical schools

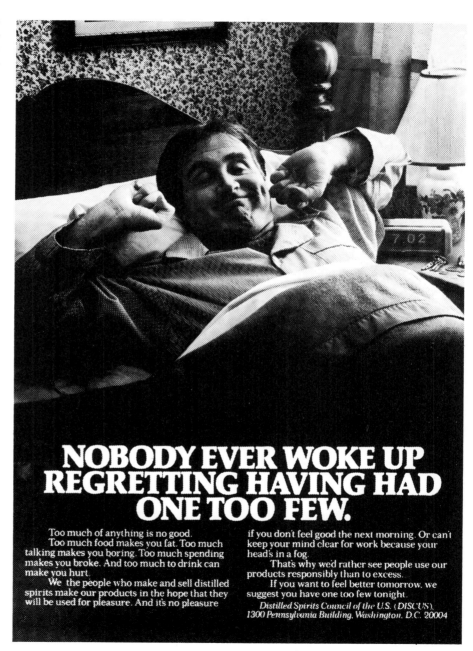

NOBODY EVER WOKE UP REGRETTING HAVING HAD ONE TOO FEW.

Too much of anything is no good.

Too much food makes you fat. Too much talking makes you boring. Too much spending makes you broke. And too much to drink can make you hurt.

We the people who make and sell distilled spirits make our products in the hope that they will be used for pleasure. And it's no pleasure if you don't feel good the next morning. Or can't keep your mind clear for work because your head's in a fog.

That's why we'd rather see people use our products responsibly than to excess.

If you want to feel better tomorrow, we suggest you have one too few tonight.

Distilled Spirits Council of the U.S. (DISCUS), 1300 Pennsylvania Building, Washington, D.C. 20004

offered some instruction in human sexuality, only 45% organized courses, and in only 42% were the courses obligatory (*1*). The situation is no better in the medical schools of Europe where, in fact, no one has even bothered to gather such data. If doctors are not being trained to have a deeper understanding of human sexuality, they cannot be expected to respond as counsellors to the needs of their patients. Sex should not move into the province of health only when there is disease or deviance; it should be a key factor in good health. We are aware today of the need for more research into the factors that affect our health, from chemicals in the environment to smoking and alcohol. We should be equally aware of the need for research into the role of sex in marriage and life. Since the studies of Masters and Johnson in the 1960s there have been changes in the attitude of society that indicate a greater tolerance and understanding, for example in relation to homosexuals. Whether new problems are emerging or old ones are simply coming to the surface, we must include positive awareness of our sexuality as part of our new approach to health (*2*).

Points for action
There are many more ways of promoting health as a way of life than outlined above. Further proposals from the official Strategy document are summarized below.

To develop awareness and provide opportunities for choice
Resources for community-based preventive programmes will have to be increased by transfer from institutional medicine. Social measures may be taken to encourage the development of satisfying family and other social networks. Research is essential to determine how far lifestyles do, in fact, affect mental and physical health.

To improve conditions that affect lifestyle and stimulate healthy behaviour
In each country every government department and every social organization, whether public or private, must make efforts to reduce unemployment, under-employment and inappropriate employment in order to ensure that everyone has a meaningful job. The health sector itself may offer more employment opportunities of a different nature if the primary health care approach is to be implemented. Occupational health services can help to reduce alienation by improving the working environment. Social networks, which are of major importance in protecting an individual's health, should be strengthened.

We must avoid taking an isolated view of social development and see each aspect as part of a whole plan of action. This takes in human ecology, and social planning for better housing and settlements, which will provide the physical framework for a mentally and physically healthy life. Conditions should be promoted which favour the development of viable local communities which can take increased responsibility for their own affairs. There should be closer integration between schools and society, with new values and services developed to facilitate the social integration of children, the elderly and the mentally and physically disabled. Closer links between the health professions and social workers as part of the new primary care teams for the community are essential. This will help lessen many of the pressures that develop when the individual has to tackle a host of different problems on his own in a system which is supposed to serve him but often seems organized to defeat him.

Research needs to be done at regional level, and in every sphere of activity, to attempt to identify conditions lying behind the choice of lifestyles and to assess the impact of changes in technologies. This is particularly true for the effect the microchip revolution and bioengineering are going to have on society, and to develop an understanding of how society and the individual can encourage the development of healthy lifestyles.

To reduce exposure to self-imposed risks
National educational efforts should be strengthened as early in life as possible to reduce individual exposure to self-imposed risks such as the abuse of alcohol and other drugs that affect the mind, smoking, unwanted pregnancy, lack of exercise, careless driving, and sexually transmitted infections.

We should raise awareness of the importance of a balanced diet and dental hygiene. The assistance of the mass media in this educational effort should be sought, and voluntary self-help groups and de-addiction clinics may be encouraged. Simultaneously, new legislative and economic measures should control the production, distribution and use of alcohol, other substances which affect the mind, and tobacco, with alternative activities for industry and trade being promoted.

In focusing on lifestyle there is, however, a real danger of appearing to be trying to create an idealized health "culture" (healthism) (*3*). Good though the intention may be to help people control their own health destiny, we must guard against placing health responsibilities on people in the belief that they will like them. There are great variations in the risks people are willing to take and the level of health care they are prepared to provide for themselves. There must therefore always be respect for individual preferences and assurance of a wide array of choice. We must at all costs avoid health programmes that involve punitive measures to achieve compliance with the "right" health behaviour.

The social cost of ill health
The following points were made by a WHO Expert Committee (*4*) with a view to gaining public support for the control of smoking. Similar points could be presented for alcoholism and several others of the new diseases.

The social cost of tobacco
Smoking entails huge economic losses which impose a burden on a national economy.

Smoking control measures should primarily be undertaken because of the deleterious health consequences of smoking. However, the economic losses lend support to the desirability of smoking control.

The collection of tobacco revenues offers no justification for delaying the implementation of measures to reduce smoking.

The world tobacco economy is dominated by a few large companies whose combined advertising budgets total about US $2000 million per year.

Tobacco production is seldom genuinely profitable for the country concerned or for individual farmers and workers and can lead to economically important negative consequences for food production. The substitution of other crops for tobacco is a vital factor in implementing smoking control in tobacco-growing countries.

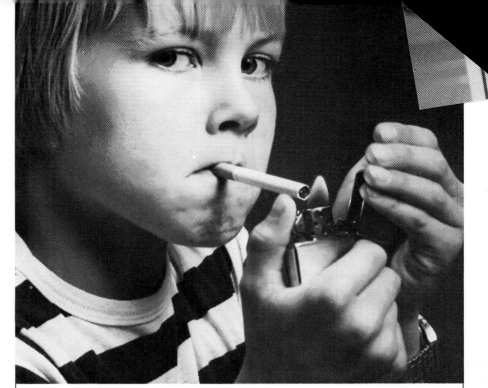

"Goodbye tobacco". In this advertisement the Danish Cancer Society promotes its anti-smoking booklet.

HVORFOR RYGER JEPPE?

Jeppe er en kvik og lærenem dreng. Derfor ryger han. Han lærer det nemlig af de voksne, som han gerne vil ligne. (Hvert 5. barn på 13 år ryger!)

Hvorfor ryger de voksne? Hvorfor ryger <u>du</u>? Det kan du finde ud af ved at læse håndbogen Farvel Tobak.

Den indeholder bl.a. 2 test-skemaer. Det ene afslører, hvorfor du ryger. Det andet afslører dine rygevaner. Farvel Tobak indeholder også gode råd, der gør det nemmere at holde op, dagbog, interviews med eks-rygere og meget mere.

Farvel Tobak udkom i forbindelse med Røgfri Dag 1980, og nu har vi genoptrykt den, fordi en stor Gallup undersøgelse viser, at den er en enestående hjælp for alle, der vil holde op med at ryge. Dine chancer, for at det skal lykkes for dig denne gang - du har jo sikkert prøvet før! - mangedobles, hvis du bestiller håndbogen Farvel Tobak. Men bestil den i dag, så vi kan nå at sende den til dig inden Røgfri Dag, mandag den 12. oktober 1981.

Sig Farvel til Tobak på Røgfri Dag mandag d. 12. oktober 1981

KRÆFTENS BEKÆMPELSE

☐ Ja tak, send mig håndbogen Farvel Tobak. Jeg vedlægger en check

FARVEL TOBAK

Navn:

Adresse:

Postnr.:   By:

OBS! I stedet for check kan giro anvendes. Indbetal min. kr. 10.- på giro 5 04 03 02, Røgfri Dag. Frederikssundsvej 123, 2700 Brønshøj. (Husk at skrive »Farvel Tobak« i rubrikken »Evt. meddelelser til beløbsmodtageren«).

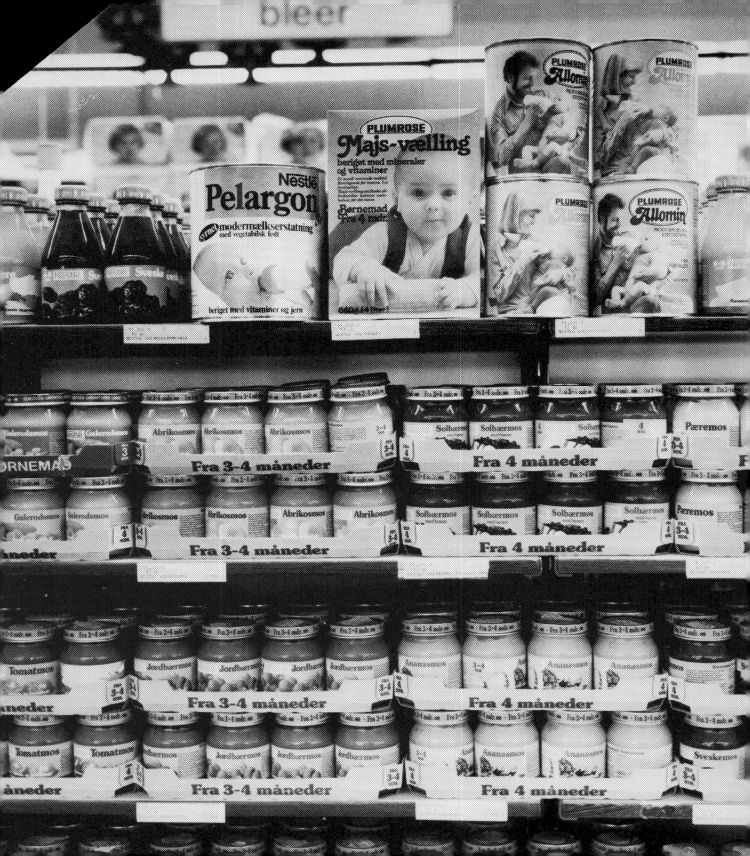

8.

The battle to prevent ill health

Belief in the powers of modern medicine has gradually reduced our confidence that, if we wish to, we can prevent or minimize the risk of falling ill. What the individual and the community can do to change their lifestyle so as not to inflict ill health on themselves has been dealt with above. However, we can also take effective action against other causes of ill health through a deeper understanding of our environment, of how we should live with it and, at times, of the measures we should take to control it. Legislation may be needed, but it must be by public demand, not imposed; we deal with that subject in the section *Legislation by public demand* on page 133. This is an integral part of the prevention of illness.

The Strategy is very specific about the various areas (poverty, perinatal care, immunization, accidents in the home and on the road, etc.) that can be tackled. This chapter will deal in turn with each of those areas (listing after each section the summary proposals from the Strategy document), but it may help to put them in perspective by first examining what we mean by "environment". The media and various groups have brought to our attention in recent years a host of different environmental issues: industrial pollution, campaigns to save wilderness areas and green spaces near our towns, efforts to save from extinction animals such as the whale and the tiger and rare birds. These issues, in a way, merely scratch the surface of the problem. The first thing to consider is the nature and effect of poverty, for an environment of poverty is the greatest creator of ill health.

Poverty

Poverty is the biggest threat to health that society faces. It is not just lack of money or wearing ragged clothing. It also means slum areas with bad housing, poor sanitation, inadequate heating and light, constant exposure to hunger and disease. All too often it means no jobs or regular income, with all the accompanying stress. It may mean poor access to good health services and inability of children to take full advantage of educational opportunities.

All these factors affect health and that is why every aspect of social development must be improved to ensure that the foundations on which health can be built are sound. Every sector of society must be involved in building those foundations. There is some justification for the view that it has been the engineers, not the doctors, who have done most to improve the health of nations in the past century because they have removed many of the sources of ill health by providing pure water, decent housing, and proper sewage disposal services.

To reduce poverty

Each country needs to examine how poverty can be reduced by such measures as social security, subsidized housing or housing allowances, land reform, tax readjustments to benefit low-income groups, and general socioeconomic development. These measures require allocation by the government of money from the public purse. The World Health Organization believes that even in economic recession the resources can be found and one area is from reduced arms spending. The World Health Assembly has said that a genuine policy of peace, détente and disarmament could and should release additional resources for such measures. At the global level, the moves to establish a just and equitable New International Economic Order, set out, for example, in the Brandt Report, would have tangible and positive results for both developing and developed countries because of their clear interdependence for mutual survival.

The importance of attacking poverty is fundamental. Specific illnesses and risks also have to be tackled. We must immunize children against disease and then keep them, through adulthood and old age, safe and well inside and outside the home.

Surviving birth

Birth is one of the most dangerous times in life that the individual faces. It may also be dangerous for the mother. It is clear that improvement should continue in the quality of services to expectant mothers so that they suffer from as little fatigue and have as natural a delivery as possible. The overmedicalization of childbirth has already been mentioned. Apart from ensuring that the whole process takes place in as normal an environment as possible (whether in the hospital or the home), we need to ensure that mother and child are close to each other after birth. The first few hours of life are very important in establishing a personal relationship between the two, and the practice of separating mother and child almost immediately militates against such a relationship. Breastfeeding has incalculable advantages in terms of mother-child contact and, for the baby, improved nutrition and defence against disease. Its displacement by artificial bottle-feeding is a trend that needs to be reversed. These approaches involve changes in social attitudes as well as medical care.

Research should also be increased on the genetic effects of modern lifestyles. As yet there is no clear evidence, but genetic changes may be transmitted to their children by smoking, drinking, and pill-taking parents. We know the effect that thalidomide and other drugs have on the foetus; the other chemicals and drugs we absorb may be storing up problems for future generations. The number of children with congenital

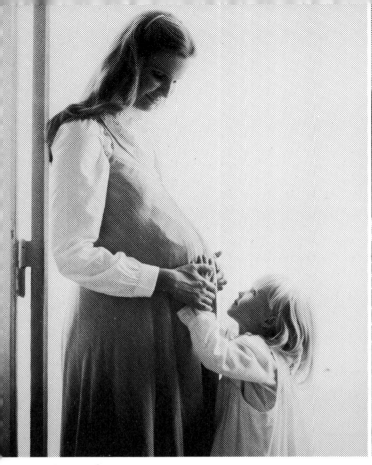

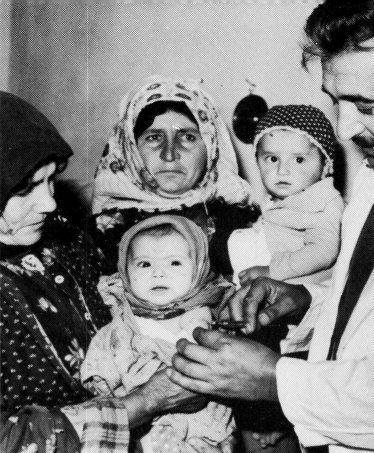

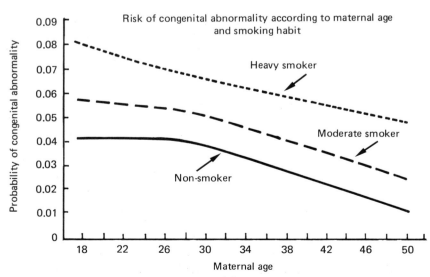

Risk of congenital abnormality according to maternal age and smoking habit

Probability of congenital abnormality

Heavy smoker

Moderate smoker

Non-smoker

Maternal age

Source: Himmelberger, D.U. et al. (*1*).

Danger in a smoke-filled womb. The probability of a mother giving birth to an abnormal baby will be higher at all ages if the mother smokes.

malformations is increasing, perhaps because we can now often take action for their survival immediately after birth. We need to find out why these malformations happen so that we can take steps to prevent them. We know that women who smoke produce smaller babies because of reduced oxygen supplies to the foetus. If alcohol can destroy the liver, what may it do to the foetus and the chromosomes that are the key to the next generations? What should a couple do if tests make it clear that they are likely to have a badly deformed child? It should be possible soon to predict such an event early in pregnancy and perhaps even before conception. This is an area involving genetic counselling, which as yet is not extensively developed but needs considerable attention.

There are growing numbers of very young mothers with special needs, but the response from social and community support systems is inadequate. The health risks are greatly magnified for such mothers and their children. The use of some contraceptives by adolescent girls may also give rise to problems and needs to be studied further. Because of the special psychological and social characteristics of adolescent sexual behaviour, adolescents often have less access to health care and family planning services, and health workers are not always prepared or able to cope with them.

To reduce perinatal risks and improve maternal and child health
At national level appropriate services for prenatal care and education and family planning should be further developed, with the support of genetic, biological, and health services research. Improved pregnancy tests should be developed and pregnant women should be encouraged to seek prenatal care as early as possible. Perinatal and maternal and child health services should ensure the early detection and permanent follow-up of defects, giving priority to high-risk families and children. More research is needed to identify toxic and other factors in the environment that cause birth defects.

Countries should cooperate to promote research that can be put into practical use in genetics and human reproduction, and to develop methods of care associated with childbearing and the early detection and control of defects and risk factors. Guidelines should be developed for the ethical use of diagnostic techniques on the foetus.

Immunization against disease

Immunization is the next vital stage after childbearing and one of the most important preventive measures we can take to protect the future health of our children. The immunized infant gets high protection in later life against some killing and debilitating diseases. In terms of suffering avoided the benefit is incalculable. The savings are also big when the cost of a vaccine is compared with the cost of treatment later in life and working time lost by the individual. The less developed countries in the Region are expanding their immunization programmes and devising new schemes for reaching people in rural areas. Their logistical problems are much more difficult than those of the industrialized countries. Vaccines need to be kept cold, from production through to use, and that can be difficult in hot climates, with irregular electricity at the main cold storage depot and no cooling facilities in the field. New portable cold boxes, using simple but advanced ideas on insulation, are helping to solve these difficulties. This work on devising new "cold chains", done through WHO, is a good example of cooperation at the practical level for primary health care. WHO's technical work on the problem with refrigerator manufacturers also shows the importance of collaboration among various sectors in society in tackling medical and logistical problems.

There is, however, a growing risk that people in the industrialized countries, who have generally been well supplied with immunization programmes, will now consider that immunization is mainly for the developing countries. This is a dangerous attitude because people will fail to ensure that the new generations of children are immunized; unvaccinated groups of children nowadays are much more exposed than previous generations as they have no resistance whatsoever. This unthinking attitude needs to be changed, and community networks have an excellent opportunity to persuade people to undergo vaccination. Parent-teacher associations should organize checks and promote vaccination, rather than merely leave it to the school authorities or the generally inadequate or nonexistent primary health care networks. The latter do seek out unvaccinated children in some countries, but what is needed is a genuine consumer demand for vaccination, not a passive waiting to be told what to do.

To reduce the incidence of preventable communicable diseases
Complete and permanent coverage of all children by expanded programmes of immunization should be achieved by 1990. The eradication of malaria and the establishment of a satisfactory surveillance system is a priority target in the infested countries. Programmes for the surveillance and control of other communicable diseases, such as viral hepatitis, tuberculosis, animal-borne diseases, parasitic diseases, gastroenteritis, and streptococcal infections, will depend on the needs of each country. Special measures will be needed to avoid the risks created by the development of tourism and international migration. Research and development work on new preventive methods, including new vaccines, must be encouraged.

At the level of the Region techniques will be developed and disseminated for the diagnosis of diseases, research on new vaccines, the identification of unconventional viruses, the adequate delivery of services, international surveillance, and the study of the spread of infection. Antimalaria activities will be coordinated, particularly to prevent the reintroduction of the disease. Regional research institutes will collaborate with the global WHO special programme for research and training in tropical diseases.

The home jungle

Accidents have become the biggest child killers in the Region, particularly in the industrialized areas and in rural areas where farming is highly mechanized. However, accidents in the home also cause much injury and death. Most of these accidents could easily be prevented,

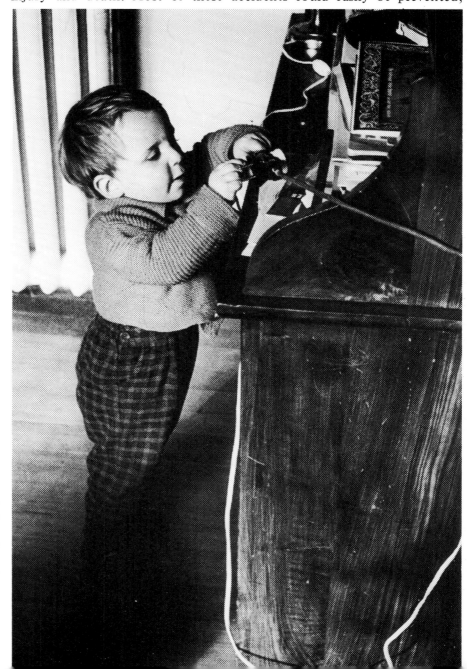

Carelessness kills. The home hides its dangers behind a deceptive facade of familiarity. Accidents are the biggest child-killers in the Region and many more accidents occur in the home than most of us realize. Parents must be taught to avoid loose electric fittings, put away medicines, keep boiling pans out of reach of children . . . in fact, always to put safety first.

particularly among the most exposed groups: children, the elderly, and those who are unwell and so take less care.

The home is a jungle that hides its dangers behind a deceptive facade of familiarity. The blind or the chairbound are normally well organized and sensitive to risks and dangers. They take care to reduce these to a minimum by adapting their surroundings to their needs and vice versa. We can learn a great deal from their routines, safety checks, and ability to depend on themselves and not on others to overcome problems. It is true that certain groups need special facilities — smooth floors and easy-to-open doors for people who cannot get around easily, alarm bells around a house or flat, or easy-to-reach telephones for the very old who need to be able to call quickly for help.

However, those of us with no apparent physical handicap are, in fact, equally at risk from falls, burns, electrocution, or fire. Gas, electricity, matches, plastic bags, slippery floors, and loose carpets are all dangers. People still keep dangerous drugs and dozens of toxic chemicals within easy reach of children. Safety in the home requires a whole routine family education. People are constantly advised on how to protect their homes against burglars, but there needs to be a much bigger effort by people to protect themselves against the dangers inside the home.

Keeping death off the road
Road accidents are now an epidemic of grave proportions. The irony is, that with all our emphasis on making sure that healthy children are born to healthy mothers and on immunizing children against the diseases that decimated them in the past, we allow them to grow up to be maimed and slaughtered on our roads. In some countries two thirds of those injured in accidents are children. However we allot the responsibility for the actual causes of accidents, there is no doubt that a double standard has developed. Government and society are happy to clamp down on vehicle manufacturers when, out of every 50 000 cars sold, one is defective and injures a pedestrian. Yet they take far too little responsibility for making sure that there are safe streets for children or extra crossings across busy roads. Poor road surfaces that cause accidents are allowed to deteriorate. Little or no provision is made for cyclists. Adolescents are given licences to drive about on fast and dangerous motorcycles. Driving offences are treated leniently.

This attitude has to be changed by public pressure so that there are more pedestrian streets, more cycle tracks, and more public transport, so that there would be less traffic on the roads. Some provision needs to be made for the growing numbers of elderly and handicapped. Driving needs to be more disciplined.

Table 6. Accidental deaths of children and young people per 100 000 in each age group, 1976

Cause of death	Age group	Germany, Fed. Rep. of		France		Italy[a]		Netherlands		Belgium		United Kingdom		Ireland		Denmark	
		M	F	M	F	M	F	M	F	M	F	M	F	M	F	M	F
Transport accidents	<1	2.0	1.7	3.0	6.5	3.1	2.1	2.2	2.3	5.0	7.0	2.0	1.2	}5.2	}3.0	2.7	8.6
	1– 4	13.1	10.1	6.6	5.2	9.4	6.4	9.3	6.7	12.1	4.8	7.2	3.8			8.8	7.0
	5–14	14.0	8.8	7.9	5.5	11.1	5.8	12.8	7.8	12.9	7.9	7.2	3.7	8.7	5.0	9.8	9.5
	15–19	82.0	23.8	53.3	18.7	43.4	11.5	42.4	15.1	69.6	20.3	44.7	10.8	40.5	13.1	65.5	18.9
	20–24	70.3	15.2	74.4	16.3	44.5	7.8	46.3	11.8	72.1	13.5	37.0	7.9	60.3	11.9	43.4	4.4
Accidental poisoning	<1	–	–	0.8	1.4	0.4	1.2	–	–	3.3	1.7	0.3	0.3	}–	}0.6	–	–
	1– 4	0.4	0.6	0.9	1.0	1.0	0.9	0.2	0.3	1.9	0.8	0.7	0.5			–	–
	5–14	0.2	0.2	0.3	0.1	0.3	0.2	–	0.1	0.9	0.3	0.2	0.2	–	–	–	–
	15–19	0.3	0.2	0.5	1.2	1.0	0.7	1.2	0.9	2.0	1.1	1.2	0.5	0.7	1.4	–	0.6
	20–24	1.3	0.4	1.1	0.8	1.3	0.6	0.7	–	2.8	2.2	2.8	0.8	1.6	–	1.0	–
Accidental falls	<1	2.7	1.7	3.0	2.3	1.6	2.4	1.1	–	5.0	1.7	2.6	2.4	}2.3	}3.7	–	2.9
	1– 4	2.0	1.7	1.7	1.1	1.3	1.5	2.2	0.5	0.8	0.4	1.6	0.6			0.7	–
	5–14	0.7	0.3	0.8	0.2	1.6	0.5	0.2	0.5	0.5	0.7	1.0	0.3	0.6	0.3	0.3	–
	15–19	1.6	0.6	2.3	0.6	3.1	0.7	0.3	0.2	1.5	0.5	1.7	0.3	1.3	1.4	0.5	–
	20–24	2.1	0.2	3.3	0.6	2.9	0.6	0.9	0.2	2.1	0.3	2.2	0.4	0.8	1.7	–	–
Accidents caused by fires and flames	<1	1.0	1.0	2.2	3.1	0.7	0.9	–	1.2	6.6	1.7	0.9	2.4	}1.2	}2.4	–	–
	1– 4	1.8	0.6	1.7	1.1	0.4	0.4	2.2	0.8	6.0	3.2	2.1	2.9			0.7	–
	5–14	0.3	0.3	0.4	0.4	0.2	0.2	0.2	0.3	0.7	0.1	0.6	0.6	1.2	0.3	0.8	–
	15–19	0.4	0.2	0.8	0.2	0.5	0.2	0.2	0.2	1.2	1.6	0.4	0.3	–	–	1.1	–
	20–24	0.8	0.3	1.3	0.7	0.5	0.1	0.3	0.2	1.3	1.1	1.2	0.4	–	–	2.1	–
Accidental drowning	<1	0.7	0.3	0.3	0.6	0.7	–	1.1	1.2	3.3	1.7	1.1	1.2	}0.6	}0.6	–	–
	1– 4	6.2	3.4	5.0	2.2	3.4	2.1	11.7	3.3	6.0	2.4	2.6	1.3			8.1	–
	5–14	2.9	0.6	2.4	0.8	3.7	0.5	3.4	0.6	1.7	0.1	1.8	0.5	2.7	0.6	1.8	0.3
	15–19	2.0	0.4	4.2	0.3	8.2	0.9	1.8	0.2	3.2	1.3	2.5	0.3	5.3	0.7	2.6	–
	20–24	3.3	0.2	5.5	0.7	5.2	0.5	2.2	0.4	3.3	1.1	1.9	0.1	6.5	–	0.5	–
All other accidents	<1	119.7	70.3	109.0	69.6	13.2	9.0	29.6	17.4	72.8	71.6	35.9	23.4	}8.1	}3.0	11.0	5.7
	1– 4	4.3	4.4	7.1	6.8	3.7	2.8	5.4	1.3	3.0	3.6	4.1	1.8			4.7	0.7
	5–14	2.4	1.1	4.0	2.1	2.3	0.7	1.4	0.4	1.6	1.0	2.2	0.5	2.7	0.6	2.3	0.8
	15–19	5.8	1.6	18.3	5.8	5.9	0.5	3.0	0.5	3.7	2.1	4.4	0.5	2.0	1.4	2.5	0.6
	20–24	6.9	1.1	23.8	4.6	6.7	0.6	3.3	0.4	4.1	2.2	5.2	0.7	6.5	–	2.1	–

[a] 1974.

Source: Statistical Office (*2*).

*As the table shows, accidents are a serious health hazard in the European
Region. The worst are traffic accidents which present the gravest danger to young
people in their 'teens and early twenties.*

To reduce accidents and their consequences

Education and information will change attitudes and reduce risk factors. A multi-sectoral approach to accident prevention will include the regulation of road construction, road traffic and pedestrian segregation, vehicle safety (including compulsory seat belt laws and the introduction of other restraining devices) and safety at work and in the home; tighter regulations on the safety of consumer goods; and the development of primary, referral and rehabilitation services for the care of the injured. Joint action by the health services and other sectors concerned in accident prevention must be promoted. In collaboration with other organizations, WHO will initiate and co-ordinate studies on the role of human and medical factors in accidents, on the cost-effectiveness of various preventive methods, on the organization of emergency medical services, and on the medical and social rehabilitation of the injured.

Safety belts save lives. Only careful driving can significantly reduce the current road accident epidemic but a quarter of the deaths in road accidents could be avoided if people always wore safety belts

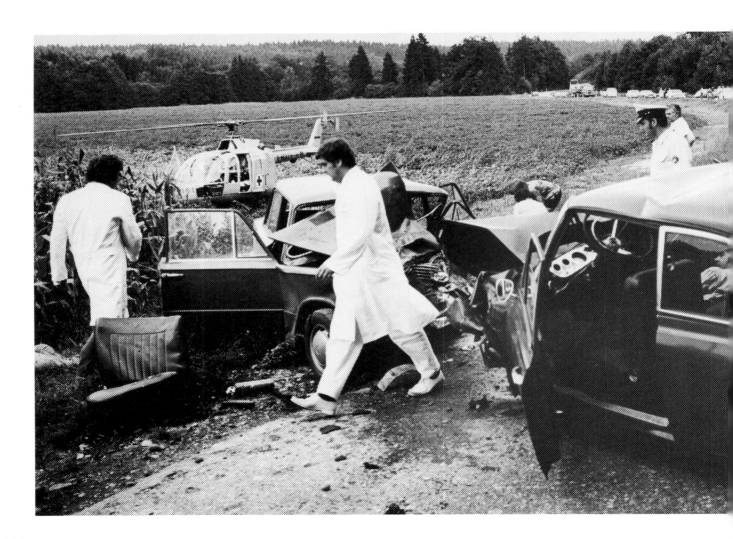

Table 7. Effect of safety belt usage laws around the world, as at 1 February 1977

Country	Effective date of law	Penalty for non-compliance	Enforcement[a]	Public information programme	Belt usage before law effective	Belt usage after law effective	Occupant fatality reduction	Occupant injury reduction
Czechoslovakia	1.1.69	max $10						
Japan	1.12.71	none	0	none		Aug 1975 8%		
Australia (all States)	1.1.72	max $20	1	yes	1971 25%	1972–1975 68–85%	1972–1974 25%	1972–1974 20%
New Zealand	1.6.72	max $200	1		May 1972 30%	1972–1975 62–83%		
France	1.7.73[b]	$10–$20	1	yes	March 1973 26%	March 1974: 64% 1975: 85% (outside cities) In city, daytime 15% night-time 30%	1975 22%	1975 32%
Puerto Rico	1.1.74	$10	0–1	yes	July 1973 3%	July 1976 25%		
Sweden	1.1.75	max $100 usual $10	1	yes	36%	March 1976 79%		
Spain	3.10.74[c]	$15						
Belgium	1.6.75	$1.50–$15.00				July 1975 92%	June – Sept 1975: 39%	June – Sept 1975: 24%
Luxembourg	1.6.75	$5.00–$12.50						
Netherlands	1.6.75	20¢–$120			Oct 1974 rural: 28% urban: 15%	June 1975 rural: 72% urban: 58%		
Finland	1.7.75	none	3	yes	June 1975 9–40%	Dec 1975 53–71%		
Norway	1.9.75	none	0	yes	Sept 1973–75 rural: 37% urban: 15%	June 1975 rural: 61% urban: 32%		
Israel	1.7.75	max $110	3	yes	June 1975 8%	Aug 1975 80% July 1976 80%		
Switzerland	1.1.76	$8	1–2	yes	May 1975 35–50%	May 1976 87–95%		
Germany, Fed. Rep. of	1.1.76	none	1	yes		Jan 1976 70–77%		
Canada (Ontario)	1.1.76	$20–$100	1	yes	Oct 1975 17%	March 1976 77% June 1976 64%	Jan – July 1976: 17%	Jan – July 1976: 15%
USSR	1.1.76	$1.50	1	none				
Canada (Quebec)	15.8.76	$10–$20	0–1	none	1.5.75 19%			

Note: blanks indicate no information available.

[a] 0 – essentially none; 1 – when motorist stopped for another purpose; 2 – strict (when observed not wearing belt); 3 – only requested to "buckle up" by officer.

[b] On roads outside city limits. 1.1.75 usage required on city roads between 10 p.m. and 6 a.m.

[c] Usage not required in cities.

Source: Ziegler, P.N. (*3*).

Poisoning the food chain

As food consumers in an industrialized society we have become accustomed to mass catering, but we have not fully understood its implications or those of the revolution in frozen foods. They are essential facts of life for vast numbers of people today, but they need constant education in their use and constant surveillance if they are to be of more benefit than harm. Food poisoning is becoming more common because of mass catering and convenience food. The reported rise in food poisoning is unfortunately only part of the picture for most cases go unreported, yet food poisoning is the second largest cause of illness in Europe today (5). Poisoning from chemical pollutants is relatively small compared with that caused by bacteria. One reason is the increase in consumption of food outside the home. Over half of all the meals eaten in Sweden each year are consumed in public places such as cafeterias and works canteens. The average stay of a worker in the kitchens of Heathrow airport, one of the world's largest, is six weeks. There are very tight checks on the catering staff, but the odds are stacked against the surveillance being adequate. Without constant vigilance airports could become the biggest and fastest exporters of food poisoning in the world. The more elaborate the food, the more handling it gets to make it look or taste better, and the higher the risk of infection from human carriers. Ironically, first-class passengers are thus more exposed to risk than those of the economy class because the latter receive more machine-prepared food. More food poisoning occurs in charter flights than regular flights, perhaps because the former are more subject to delays and food is kept too long or is taken on board in hot countries where inadequate refrigeration may be a problem.

Table 8. Infectious enteric diseases in Europe, 1973–1979[a]					
	Year				
	1973	1974	1975	1976	1977
Salmonellosis	20 406	16 053	60 115	81 586	47 282
Other gastrointestinal infections	143 422	123 791	162 284	605 556	583 056

[a] As notified to the World Health Organization.

Source: Velimirovic, B. (4).

There has been an explosion in cases of food poisoning in Europe in recent years.

The great international movements of tourists are also a major cause of infection. Those who travel to areas where water and sanitation facilities are poor act as international carriers of disease. They may go to areas where they are not resistant to the local bacteria connected with food. The local population may not only be resistant — they may also prepare their food in traditional ways that reduce the risk of infection. The tourists look for their own kind of food, which may not be suitable for the different climate and may be cooked in conditions favouring infection. Alternatively, they ask for cold food, fruit or salads, which present a grave risk unless properly prepared.

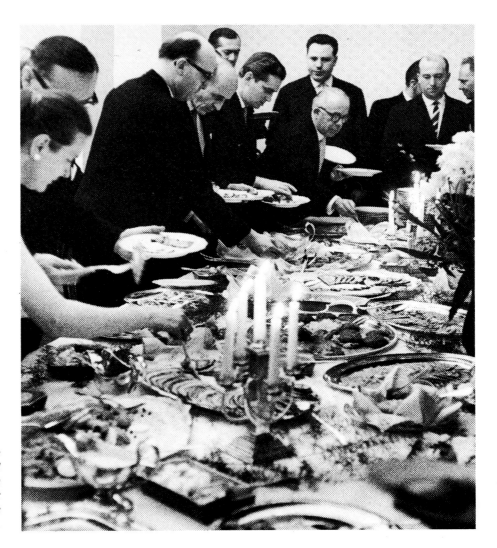

The fancier the food, the greater the risk: food prepared for an elaborate reception is handled many times to make it look decorative, increasing the chances of it becoming infected.

Catering jobs quite often, too, rank among the lowest paid, and many catering workers live in an environment not conducive to good health. Thus, they risk infecting others by the food they prepare and serve.

Generally, food is no longer processed locally. The consumer nowadays in the European Region as often as not buys plastic-wrapped products, often frozen or pre-cooked, which may have come from the other side of the world. This makes the need for proper enforcement of internationally agreed food controls important. It will be discussed further on pages 133–135, in the chapter on *The role of politics*, as an example of legislation for health.

Good food, good diet
Giving young children wholesome food and a balanced diet protects them from illness and ill health. The poorly-fed child is in far more danger than the well-fed from infections that cause diarrhoea (the biggest killer of the 17 million children in the world who die every year, most of them in the developing world). In an urbanized society additives and preservatives in food are needed, but far more time and money must be spent on research into their effects and into those of unnecessary and perhaps harmful colouring agents. It is possible, without going in for fads, to produce foods more naturally, but the cooperation of producer and consumer will be needed.

To promote balanced nutrition and safe food
The main thrust should be on education and information to promote balanced nutrition and avoid obesity as well as malnutrition, particularly in infants and adolescents. The production of adequate food should be encouraged, and policies devised to ensure that low-income groups can get enough food. Food safety services should be developed; breastfeeding should be promoted. There should be a common approach among ministries who have any relations with, or control over, the food industry (sales, pricing, production, taxing, inspectorates, etc.) to control it with a view to improving food quality and safety. Changing patterns of feeding and nutrition in children, adolescents, and vulnerable groups in industrialized and industrializing societies must be monitored. Health education models in this field will be developed. Attention will also be devoted to research, information, education, and training in food safety services, with particular emphasis on mass catering.

Polluting the planet
We have created new threats to our environment and we must now develop a new approach so as to be able to combat them effectively. Much worse than the dramatic examples that fill the headlines is the pollution that occurs insidiously in our everyday environment. Thus, while most air pollution control and testing is carried on out of

doors — the very place where people spend the least part of their time — the family lives in a home insulated against every breath of air from outside (6), where the fitted carpet harbours a host of bacteria and has perhaps been stuck down with toxic glue, the father suffers from the strains of his work, the elder son smokes, the daughter produces ear-splitting sounds from a hi-fi system, and the mother takes tranquillizers in glasses of soft water with the natural salts removed and prepares shellfish from a polluted sea for the family to eat. It is the effect of combinations of factors such as these that we have not really started to understand.

Noise is another important hazard that we now recognize in our lives. For example, more than 8 million people among the United Kingdom's 56 million suffer from a significant loss of hearing, and 2 million need aids (7,8). An oil rig in the North Sea may not be the only place where ear mufflers are needed. There are many industries in which noise in the workplace is doing unrecognized and preventable damage, but there is probably more ear damage done in Europe in discotheques and in children's bedrooms from sound equipment than from anything else, though that caused by the motorcycles of the young must run it close.

Again, between 200 and 1000 new chemical products arrive on the market every year. The companies who produce and the consumers who either demand or are persuaded that they need them could play a more positive role in deciding exactly what is really needed, and the risks must be thoroughly assessed. We are also moving into the era of micro-electronics and bioengineering, which could dramatically alter our working and social life. It is essential that there should be planned research so that we do not find ourselves trying to patch up the social and health effects of these revolutions in our lives, otherwise the cost may be enormous in human and financial terms.

We shall never understand the effects of all the good and bad environmental stimuli unless we take an overall view while looking into the detail. We must also avoid making people feel, through our lifestyles and preventive approaches, that health is an unacceptably sterile ideal. That is why we must all be involved in deciding what are acceptable risks, bearing in mind that we may be storing up long-term effects we may regret. We must react with full awareness to our environment and make greater use of environmental impact assessment, i.e., the technique of assessing the impact on the environment of major industrial projects and land developments and of the micro-climates in which we spend much of our lives.

To reduce environmental risks

Chemical, physical and biological hazards, including noise and radiation, should be identified and controlled through the implementation of technical, legislative, administrative and economic measures, and health education to increase general awareness of environmental risk factors.

Intercountry programmes will establish monitoring systems to identify and assess environmental hazards, develop and disseminate information control methods and technical, legislative, administrative and economic measures for environmental protection and safety, and to promote staff training.

To provide safe water and sanitation

Safe drinking-water and sewage disposal systems for all should be achieved by 1990 as part of the global plan of the World Health Assembly and the United Nations International Drinking-Water Supply and Sanitation Decade. To achieve this target, technologies will have to be identified and disseminated to solve the remaining problems of smaller communities, in rural, arctic and arid areas, and in poorly equipped urban areas. Minimum standards of housing hygiene should be established.

The identification of resources will be one of the first priorities up to 1990. Emphasis should be on the needs of countries in southern Europe, where cooperation with the World Bank, the United Nations Development Programme (UNDP), the United Nations Environment Programme (UNEP), and other agencies will be strengthened. Problems of housing and urban development will also be given high priority, as well as the introduction of appropriate technologies for development in remote areas.

The factory worker's food prepared in stainless steel vats like these is safer. But because of the thousands who may eat from the same kitchen, one infection can lead to many more cases of gut trouble.

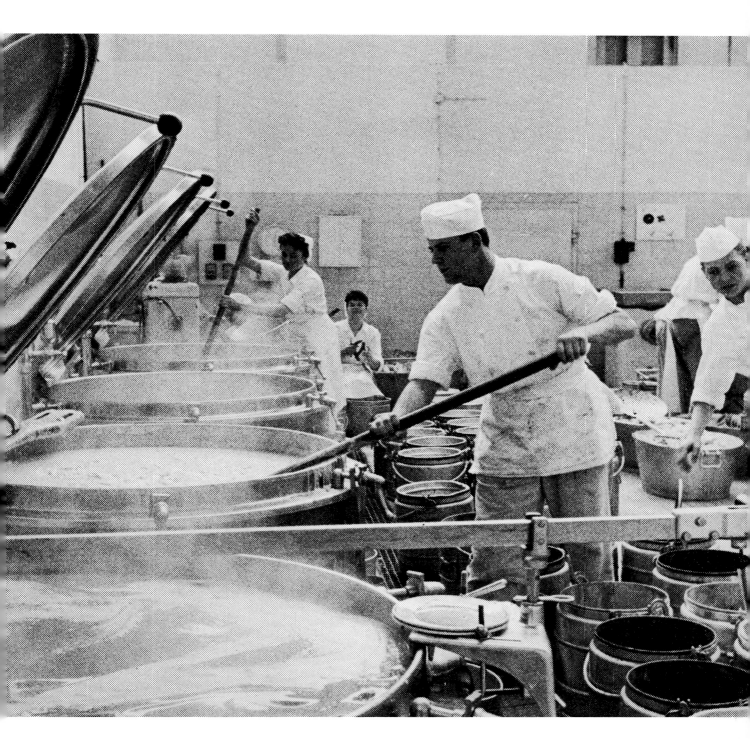

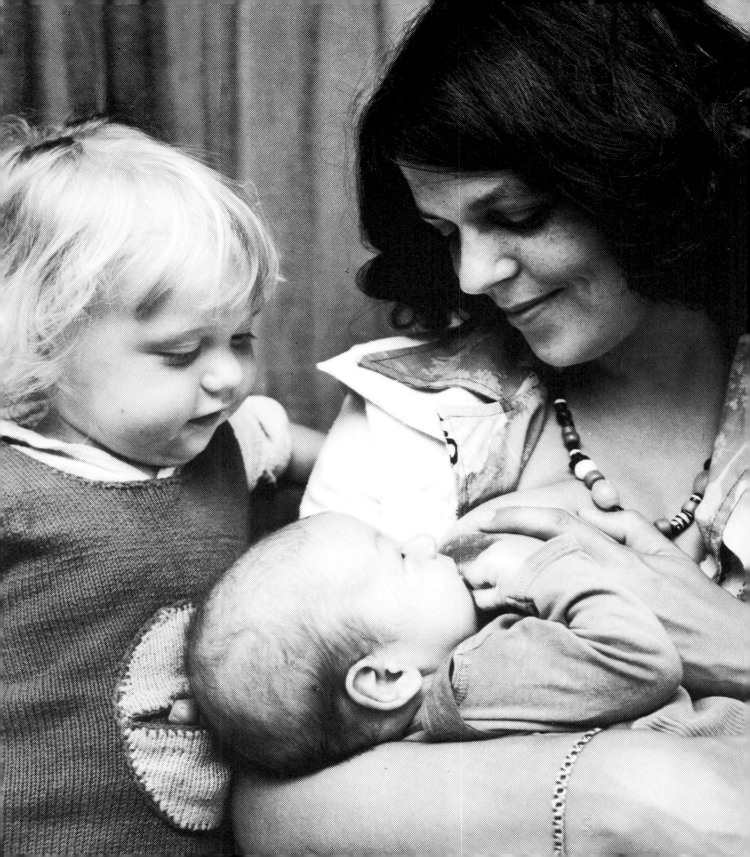

9.

Community care
means people

Community care systems using primary health care as a key were discussed earlier. The essence of that care is not a return to a primitive state, but the exact opposite. If people get the right care at the right time, we save them from being left until they have eventually to crawl, or be carried, further into a system where preventing or reducing risk is no longer an option and the only solution is advanced "care". An example of a critical situation is a heart attack. The present trend is towards getting the patient to the nearest hospital as fast as possible. Studies have shown, however, that the patient's knowledge that he will be sent immediately to hospital often means that a doctor is not called in time. In many instances, too, the doctor has come to feel safer leaving the whole operation in the hands of the specialized emergency system. The development of highly mobile, cheap, sophisticated equipment, however, is feasible. In the hands of the local doctor or other trained members of new primary health care teams, such equipment could have a much better effect at far less cost than hundreds of intensive care or coronary units in hospitals.

Home can be best

A considerable amount of research is being done on caring for heart attack victims at home after brief hospitalization, or even without hospitalization at all. The evidence seems to suggest that in many cases this is better than staying in hospital. If good home care with proper guidance is made possible, the patient benefits by being in his own surroundings and the pressure on hospitals is relieved. It has long ago been shown that, with the availability of better drugs, outpatient treatment of tuberculosis is more cost-effective than sending patients to a sanatorium. Other areas can undoubtedly be found where, with proper support and provision for care, home can be best.

The principle of the most suitable care at the right time involves a complete rethinking of our approach. We need the skills of doctors to effect the education of people, to detect problems early, and to make sure that the system of referral is effective, speedy, and relevant. There are enormous blockages in hospital systems because people with minor ailments fail to get help early. Often, after weeks or months of waiting to see a specialist, the elderly person needing a new hip joint may have to join a long queue before being operated on. In the meantime, the blockages affect the whole system and result in immense unnecessary suffering. The old person gradually goes downhill while waiting for the operation, becoming less and less able to fend for himself.

Provision for the weak

Provision for the weaker groups is just as important. The mentally ill and the elderly should be regarded as integral parts of society, not to be put to one side because they have become social nuisances. Fine words will not achieve this change. There have been marked advances in the integration of drug addicts and alcoholics into the community, but perhaps too much of the integration has been accomplished in the face of resistance from society and those who allocate the funds. The institutionalized mentally ill face a bigger problem of reintegration into the community than any other group because they are part of a formidably well established system. An example of what can be done for the mentally ill will show how far we could go in assisting the integration of other weaker groups.

Freeing the prisoners of mind and body
The story of the reform of the mental hospital in Trieste is too long to detail here, but it symbolizes the work that can and must be done (1). It was based on a fundamental shift from the padlocked institution to the caring therapeutic role of the community.

In 1968 there were 1270 patients, mainly compulsorily detained, in the *Ospedale Psichiatrico Provinciale,* including the mentally ill and mentally retarded. Many of the patients had first been taken to a general hospital casualty department. There, they had been examined and, if necessary, compulsorily committed to the mental hospital by a physician without psychiatric training whose recommendation was countersigned by a police officer. The changes made by the director, Professor Basaglia, meant that, by 1971, 220 beds had been vacated by discharging patients and 230 of the remaining 1050 patients had been designated as voluntary. Those who remained were moved into mixed wards and more were given voluntary status. Patients who had worked for the psychiatric hospital for long hours, getting only 600 lire and 800 cigarettes a month, were formed into a cooperative. They now get outside work from schools and private individuals and the minimum rate of pay is 1380 lire per hour. The cooperative runs at a profit, which goes into a pension fund.

Since many elderly, disabled, long-stay patients could not be discharged, they were given the status of "guests", which entitled them to certain social security benefits and removed certain social disadvantages. The wards and former staff accommodation were transformed into group apartments on the hospital site. Despite staff strikes and court cases, the changes went on and the discharges continued. When a long-standing proposal to rebuild the hospital was brought up again in 1975, it was decided that rebuilding would not be necessary – the hospital would not be needed because three district health centres opened in 1974 were working and doing their job well. With the completion of the system of community centres and teams in 1977, hospital admissions,

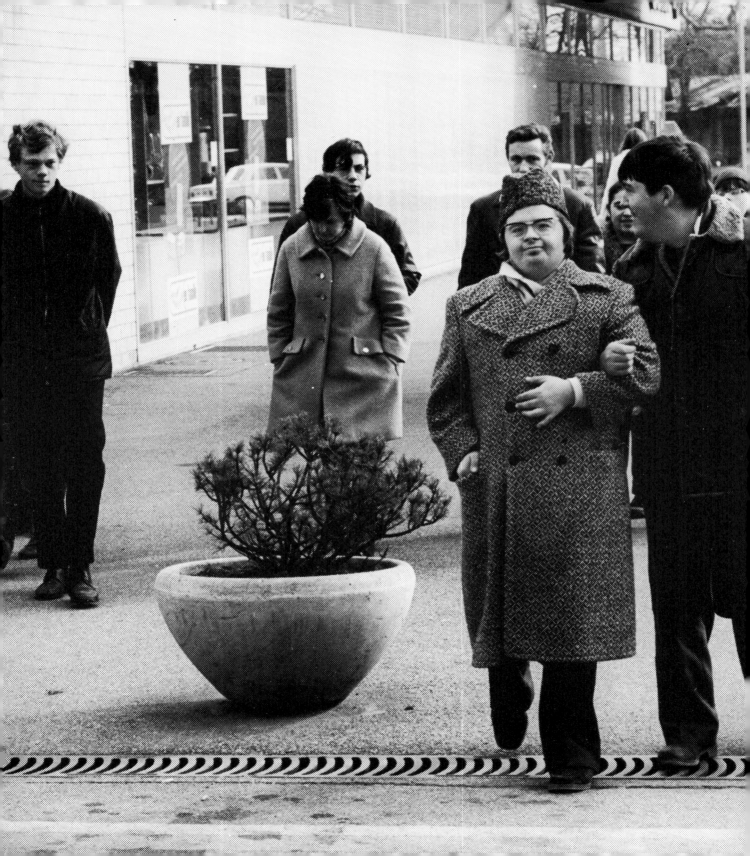

which had already been reduced, were discontinued. There are many questions surrounding the whole scheme but it is likely that most of these questions would never have arisen had it not been necessary to almost drag the public and the health professions to a realization of how wrong things had been. With the full cooperation of the community from the start, other such ventures would suffer none of the difficulties of Trieste.

Self-reliance

Apart from the real health benefits of self-reliance, the involvement of the community is an active way of removing the mystique of medicine. The spread of self-management for people with colostomies and similar disabilities or limitations means a growing ability to cope with conditions that would have been unthinkable for many in the past without hospital care. It should also mean that people need to stay in hospital for shorter periods. (2)

If relatives and friends know and accept as normal the needs of diabetics, it is no great step for them to accept the needs of heart-risk patients, or to operate personal blood-pressure gauges or other appropriate, simple equipment that could be developed with new technology. We should no more allow the elderly person to degenerate and become a helpless dependant than we should leave the heart attack victim to die; instead, we should see their problems early and design life around them so that they can continue to cope.

Specific points on community care in the Strategy document include the following.

To provide equal access to appropriate health care
Community-based health systems should be established or developed. In these, primary health care will be the central function, backed up by hospital services, including facilities for referral of patients to more specialized institutions and for supervision, guidance, and logistical support. Resources for national health services, at the moment concentrated in cities and on specialist services, should be redistributed to ensure the accessibility of acceptable services to all groups of the population. A particular effort is needed to ensure the quality of care: that services are far more human, personal and relevant to real community and family needs. This requires the involvement of other organizations and groups related to health, a maximum of self-reliance and participation by the individual and the community, and a new understanding of the role of health workers. The health team, and particularly general practitioners, nurses and midwives, will have to be trained and retrained in the spirit of full community care. In addition, in order to promote the full participation of local communities, health information and education of both the population and the health professions must be an important part of the system. Putting the system into effect should be a priority in underserved areas, and particularly declining inner city areas and rural areas with low populations.

To provide special care for high-risk groups

Gaps should be filled by ensuring special services to underserved and particular risk groups. However, it is essential that these services are integrated into the health system and social networks. Children and adolescents should be reached through family health, school health, dental, and mental health services. Special consideration should be given to the elderly and to the rehabilitation of the disabled when planning and implementing health and social services. The elderly and disabled should be actively involved in this through appropriate social networks and the powerful framework of community care. Thought should be given to promoting dignified and appropriate care for the dying. There is a recent and growing awareness that the work of hospices for the dying has much to teach us in this area.

We must also encourage research between countries on the cost-effectiveness of services including self-care and self-help approaches, with studies on special aspects of delivering health services in arctic and arid areas.

To reduce the effects of chronic and degenerative diseases

Technical and educational methods should be developed for the early detection, diagnosis, timely treatment, and rehabilitation of these diseases, making appropriate use of self-help and self-care approaches. Research to identify further environmental, genetic, and behavioural risk factors should be accompanied by the development of appropriate preventive measures, involving the community in the attack on social risk factors. Medical, social, and economic rehabilitation services should be developed, and sectoral programmes integrated into service delivery systems.

Countries will be encouraged to exchange expertise in medical research and to develop research on the study of the spread of disease and methods for the prevention and early detection of chronic diseases, based on the involvement of the community and the individual. Special attention will be given to the development of pilot schemes for primary prevention, and research into cost-effective care and rehabilitation services, and the acceptability of the least expensive, effective treatment plans.

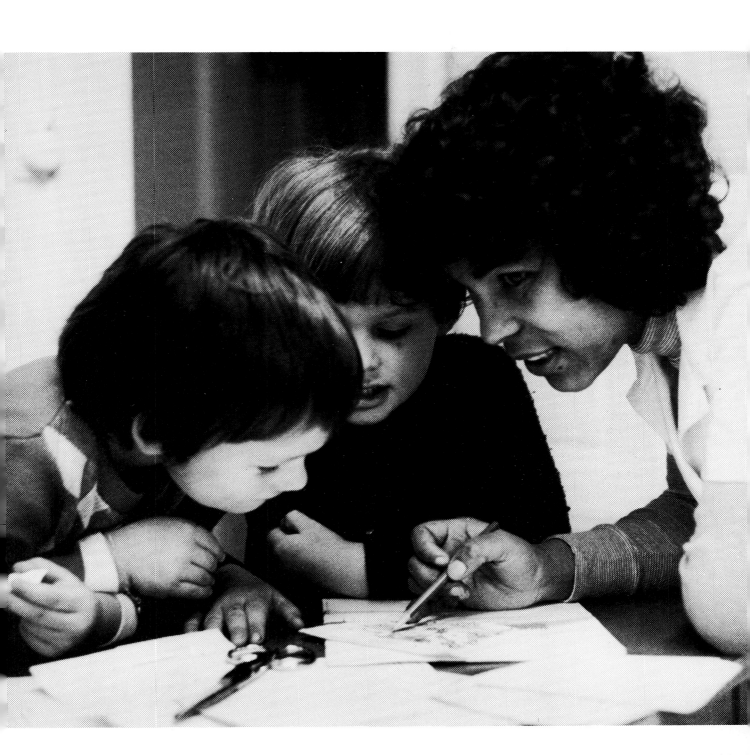

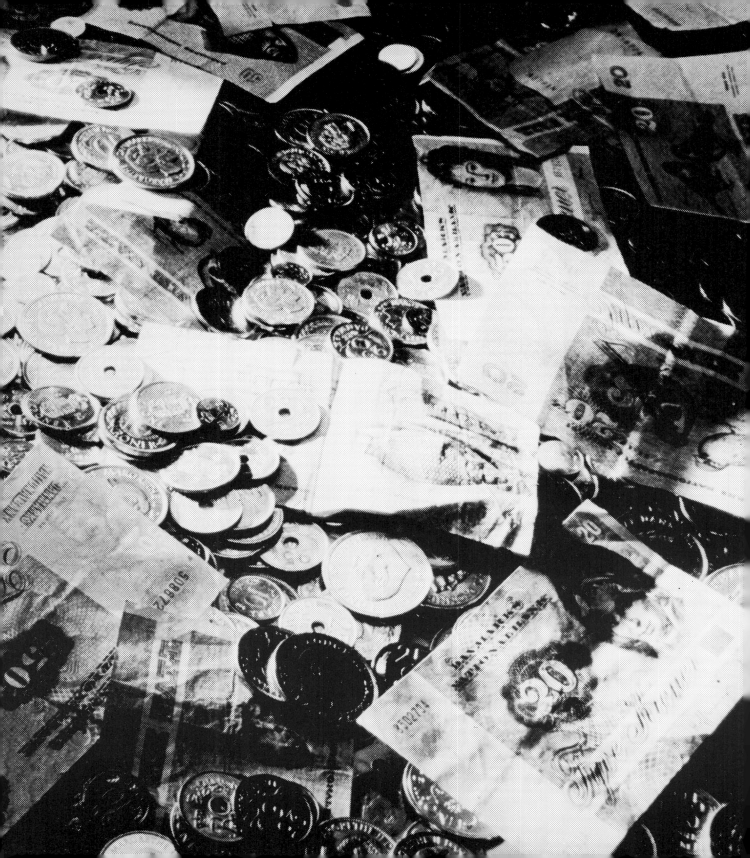

10.

Value for money

The politician who succeeds in raising the "health consciousness" of the people will undoubtedly go down as one of the shrewdest persons in political history. The economic benefits of a true strategy for health for all are enormous. A nation that is healthy is more productive. If people participate in a community care health system, with prevention of ill health as a way of life, the cost of curing people from self-imposed illness will fall dramatically. In the face of recession no nation at present can afford to continue pouring resources into high-technology hospitals that can meet only 10–20% of its health needs.

Money alone is not enough

A simple cut in allocations is not enough: what is needed is a shift of resources to produce a new emphasis. This is a strategic decision that will lead to greater effect and more benefits. There is no doubt that the training of the personnel needed, the provision of more home care, and the equipment of health care centres will mean substantial outlays. This will not be pouring good money after bad, however – it will be an investment in the community: in health centres and health promotion campaigns, not in "disease palaces".

Improving the promotion of health so that it is effective at the level of the community will release resources all the way through the health system and make more available for vital services. In time it will mean that, as more and more people stay healthy or are cured earlier when ill, the more sophisticated levels within the system will be freed from trying to cope with large numbers of very ill patients. Thus, the queues of people waiting for operations will diminish and the specialists will be able to give adequate time and attention to the patients under their care.

Some streamlined services

More healthy lifestyles will mean fewer people suffering from disorders of the heart. Those who develop them will be detected much more quickly through the primary health teams. The teams could have new, cheap, efficient, and safe equipment, shared with the patient and relatives, to do check-ups regularly at home or in a community centre and ensure appropriate home care when danger threatens. The effect would be to relieve hospital outpatient and casualty departments and cardiologists, and costs would be cut at the expensive hospital stage of the care system. As the numbers of heart cases diminished, the resources released could be channelled into improving the system so that the same quality of health care was available to all when needed. Similarly, hospital funds and facilities would be released so that highly specialized heart surgery could receive a proper allocation of resources. Research into the causes of cardiovascular disease, as of other conditions, would also be given proper support. It would not have to rely constantly on philanthropic benefactors because regular funds were being drained away in inappropriate care systems.

There are more innovative ways of getting immediate care to heart attack victims, and high technology can be appropriate and may not necessarily be expensive. One can already put a simple monitoring device on the chest of a patient who is known to be at risk and has suffered an attack. This device can then be plugged into the telephone to link the patient electronically to an expert at a central monitoring centre who can diagnose and direct while help arrives. There are professional and other barriers to be overcome with this kind of approach but, if we are able to use the 'phone to buy a washing machine with a credit card without moving from our armchair, it would seem common sense to use the same system to stop ourselves dying!

Greater home care of the elderly or the mentally ill needs more resources at the local level, which should save expenses on centralized institutions. If elderly persons can easily attend a local centre when needing more than a home check-up by relatives, their life will be improved.

New health for all involves a steady advance of community care, more healthy lifestyles for individuals, and prevention programmes. To the effects in human terms of less alcohol, fewer cigarettes, and more protection against disease through immunization, the economists will add the economic effects of less illness at work and at school.

Gilt-edged investment

Within the Strategy there must be programmes to identify causes of ill health and seek ways and means of removing them. Not all diseases can be combated in the way WHO eradicated smallpox, but that disease provides a dramatic illustration of the economic benefits a successful campaign can bring. As smallpox is spread by people only, it was possible to launch a military-style surveillance programme to track down individual carriers and vaccinate all those with whom they had been in contact. WHO masterminded the operation, but the real work was done by tens of thousands of field workers throughout the world tracking down every case of smallpox (1,2). As a result of the campaign, the developing countries effectively gave the developed world one of the biggest returns on an investment ever known. Smallpox was officially declared eradicated in May 1980, two years after the last case was located in the Horn of Africa. This means that vaccination everywhere can be stopped and that travellers no longer need vaccination certificates. The savings throughout the world are estimated to be US $1000 million annually (see box).

> Already the international community is starting to collect part of the health legacy — and it is likely to be huge — that smallpox eradication will bequeath. Calculations indicate that in the post-smallpox era a sum of nearly US $1 000 million annually will be released . . .
>
> The cost to the world of a disease like smallpox included production or purchase of vaccine, maintenance of vaccination programmes, the treatment of vaccination complications, spending to maintain national surveillance and frontier controls, and the cost involved in handling the emergencies caused by sudden outbreaks. Thus, in the United Kingdom, an outbreak sparked by an imported case in 1961 involved a bill for an estimated US $3.6 million. United States experts calculate that smallpox protection was costing the American taxpayer about US $150 million a year — or about half the total cost of the global eradication programme . . . (3)

The same approach is beginning to be applied to preventing the millions of cases of unnecessary damage to sight caused by vitamin deficiencies, easily preventable eye infections, or cataracts, which can be removed by a simple and cheap operation. The benefits would be enormous because of the approximately 40 million people in the world whose sight is impaired in one way or another. The involvement of eminent blind people in the campaign at international level is a classic instance of how the disadvantaged in society can play a full role in tackling world problems.

Advanced technology for the people

Some say that the possible future use of modern miniaturized electronic equipment in the home to deal with health problems originally tackled in the high-technology hospital will raise an even greater barrier between the rich and poor parts of the Region. This is an assumption which may spring too easily from an industrialized lifestyle which arrogantly assumes that others cannot afford, could not use, or do not need technology, high or low. However, we are talking about cost-effective technology. The battery-operated transistor radio can be found in the most remote nomadic encampments within the Arctic Circle or in the deserts of the Sahara. The transistor revolutionized mass communications worldwide and made that dangerous commodity, information, available to all, even in the poorest village. Now that miniaturized electronic equipment has become cheap, there is no reason why a primary health care worker should not be able to carry with him a microchip-based, low cost, mass-produced blood analysis machine for malaria or a digital display blood-pressure gauge. High technology does not have to be expensive — it needs to be appropriate. Designers of high-technology equipment should start thinking about everyday use by the people, not just the hospital market.

Microchips for everyone. The marvels of the microchip can be used to bring health to all the different peoples of the European Region of WHO, from Reykjavik in Iceland to Vladivostok in the USSR and from the wastes of the Arctic to the deserts of the Sahara. Because the microchip allows us to make many devices small and cheap, it will not only serve those in our cities who have immediate access to high-technology hospitals but reach also those in the most remote of rural communities

The following is a summary, from the Strategy document, of the areas that must fall within the scope of cost-effectiveness in order to provide better service in health.

To improve cost-effectiveness and quality of services
Care programmes should ensure a high quality of care, equity and continuity, while at the same time realizing the principle of the lowest effective level of care. Models of such health care programmes should be developed. Professional review systems should be encouraged and professionals should be made responsible for cost containment and reducing uneconomical procedures. Care programmes should increase the level of communication and the sharing of responsibilities among the various categories of personnel.

Intercountry collaboration in health services research and development will be strengthened, with special emphasis on cost-effectiveness. Information concerning professional review systems will be exchanged. A regional network of national institutions will be used to improve knowledge of existing and future problems, assess present and newly developed technologies, develop techniques for assessing cost-effectiveness, and test model health care programmes.

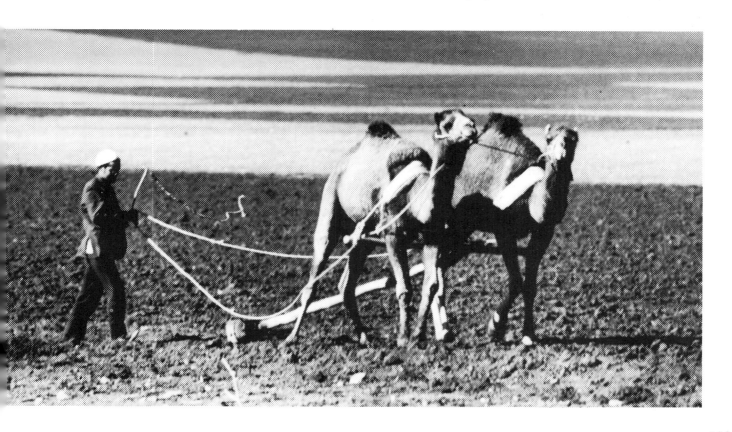

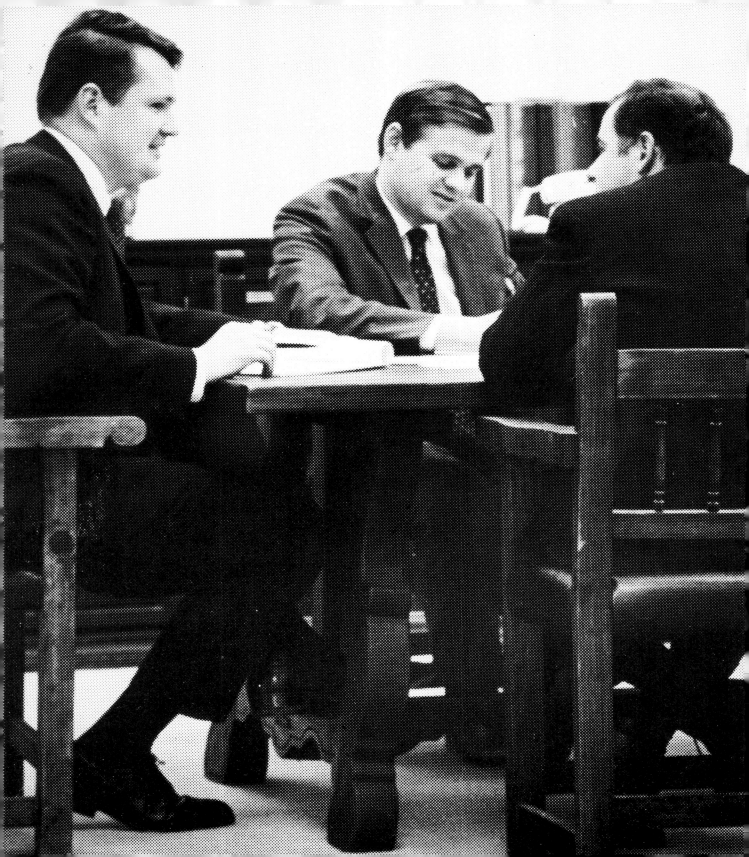

11.

The role of politics

The political implications of the Strategy are far-reaching. They include a fundamental shift in social attitudes, an important change in relationships inside the medical profession, and the reallocation of resources: people, money, and equipment. The Strategy represents a challenge, however, not a threat. By definition, community care is a people's movement, established not on a narrow but on the broadest of political bases.

Although heads of government and ministers take the lead, they respond to public pressure. The creation of local, regional, and national councils or commissions of citizens, in which women play a powerful role, should be seen as an addition to the political process. Such councils should have the power to effect change and promote progress. They should not be regarded as another consultative body whose proposals gather dust on shelves.

Community care involves decentralization and, therefore, greater control over local affairs by local people and their representatives. Too many government health strategies have, in fact, produced networks of services that are more and more remote from those they are supposed to serve. Full political support must be given to ensuring that community care does not fall into that trap.

Cyclists demonstrate to demand road space. The successful cyclists' lobby in Denmark has helped create many miles of paths, segregating cyclists from motor traffic. The resulting increase in safety has saved many lives as well as encouraging many more people to use bicycles, the healthiest form of transport.

CONSUMER GROUPS

Within the new decision-sharing structure much greater advantage must be taken of the talents that many existing health or social groups have to offer. These include special skills such as those available in Alcoholics Anonymous, spina bifida groups, and groups for the elderly. They also include those of other bodies such as the educational wing of trade unions and professional associations of architects or businessmen.

Pressure groups have a key role to play because of their knowledge, whether they are consumer associations or the environment lobby in all its forms. Ramblers, cyclists, joggers and mountaineers, active sports enthusiasts and those who take their daily constitutional — all need to convert their enthusiasms into political weapons for change.

MINISTRIES, PEOPLE, AND THEIR REPRESENTATIVES

In governments the health minister must come to be regarded as one of the most important. This is not because the health ministry must be given most money; indeed, full awareness of the health aspect in every sector of the economy will eventually save the nation money. The reason is that the Strategy proposed will inaugurate a process of change that will affect the entire nation.

Politicians who are not executive members of a government or who are Members of the European Parliament or the Assembly of the Council of Europe all have a role to play. The time has come for them to demand, on behalf of their constituents and the pressure groups, far more detailed data from civil servants to find out what has gone wrong and how to change it. Representatives with high unemployment in their area must be particularly concerned, for they are living with a health hazard that will definitely take its toll within a few years.

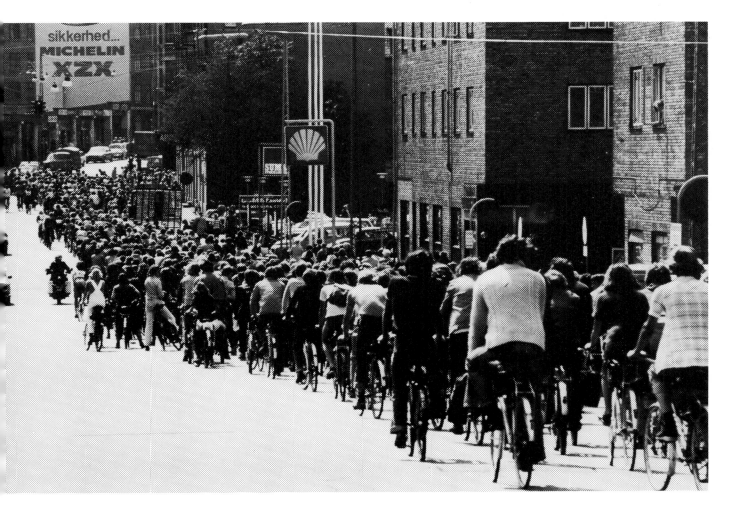

THE LEVERS OF CHANGE — MANPOWER AND PLANNING

Health manpower is essential to any successful programme of action and needs to be responsive to the fundamental shift in direction that is required. The task is complex; if a country lacks the people to carry it out it must, as a priority, create the manpower to carry out the political decisions that emerge from local and national debate about community care.

The impersonality of health services has, in the past, alienated the public from those who work in and manage the services. The latter, too, have suffered from the inflexible rules and regulations with which they have been surrounded. Since it is intended that community care should spread across the whole range of public life, and not simply health ministry officials and medical personnel, a new element of cooperation on both sides needs to develop. Careful planning for a system of community care should bring officials and administrators at all levels back into genuine consultation and greater contact with the public and put an end to rigid bureaucracy. It is worth repeating here that civil servants in the health ministries should follow training courses which have an overlap where possible with those for the medical profession. It is also important that officials from other ministries such as housing, sanitation, road transport, or energy should be provided with courses on health. This would give them an overview of public life and of how health relates to most areas, and thus lead to greater cooperation.

The Strategy document, well aware of this kind of problem, offers the following general summary of how the overall process should be tackled.

At country level health planning and management should be flexible so that national planning is more concerned with general principles, the development of strategies, coordination and resource allocation, while local levels are given more responsibility for adapting principles to the characteristics of the community. Participation of providers and the population in planning is essential to ensure positive cooperation in implementing plans. Special care should be taken to see that women are included in the determination and implementation of health policy and care at the local and national levels, not only as beneficiaries but also as participants in the processes.

The countries will have to develop or refine their management tools, particularly in planning, programming, evaluation and information systems. Health development networks, based on existing institutions, could provide national facilities for planning, management, research and training. The health administration will have to be adapted, and legislation may be needed, to strengthen the coordinating role of departments of health and other elements of the national network, and to increase their participation in socioeconomic development. National health councils or similar bodies will play an essential role by ensuring a multisectoral approach.

Table 9. Imports and exports of sulfur emissions[a] in 1974
(dry plus wet; 10^3 tons of sulfur)

Receivers	Emitters																	Total received from all areas	Total emitted to all areas[b]
	Participants in OECD study											Surrounding areas							
	Austria	Belgium	Denmark	Germany, Fed. Rep. of	Finland	France	Netherlands	Norway	Sweden	Switzerland	United Kingdom	Czechoslovakia	German Dem. Rep.	Italy	Poland	Other areas	Unattributed		
Participants in OECD study:																			
Austria	60	6	0	40	0	20	2	0	0	5	20	20	20	30	7	20	30	300	221
Belgium	0	100	0	20	0	30	5	0	0	0	30	1	4	0	0	1	10	200	499
Denmark	0	1	60	6	0	3	1	0	2	0	10	1	6	0	2	2	10	100	312
Germany, Fed. Rep. of	8	60	7	700	0	100	40	0	2	7	100	20	80	7	10	10	90	1 250	1 964
Finland	0	2	8	10	100	4	2	2	30	0	10	7	30	0	20	80	70	400	274
France	2	40	1	50	0	600	10	0	0	6	100	5	20	30	2	30	150	1 000	1 616
Netherlands	0	10	1	10	0	10	60	0	0	0	0	1	4	0	1	0	10	150	391
Norway	0	4	8	10	1	9	4	30	9	0	60	3	10	0	5	4	100	250	91
Sweden	0	7	30	30	10	10	6	6	100	0	40	8	50	0	20	30	100	500	415
Switzerland	1	2	0	7	0	20	1	0	0	30	10	2	1	6	1	2	20	100	76
United Kingdom	0	8	2	10	0	20	4	0	0	0	800	2	9	0	2	1	100	1 000	2 883[c]
Surrounding areas:																			
Czechoslovakia, German Dem. Rep., Italy, Poland and other areas	60	60	80	400	40	200	40	9	50	10	600	900	1 300	900	1 000	4 500	1 000	11 000	—
Total emitted to above areas	100	300	200	1 300	150	1 000	200	40	200	60	1 800	1 000	1 500	1 000	1 100	4 600	1 900	17 000	—

[a] Numbers are rounded to the nearest significant figure for individual countries, and accurate to within about ± 50%. The totals have been rounded separately except for the last column to the right.

[b] 1973 data from OECD Emissions Survey.

[c] Includes 80 $\times$ 10^3 tons of sulfur from Ireland.

Source: OECD Observer (1).

Poisoning each other. The many tons of pollutants, released into the air by various countries in Europe, rain down from the skies onto their European neighbours. We can protect ourselves against such health risks only by international cooperation.

A HEALTH POLICY FOR EUROPE –
INTERNATIONAL COOPERATION

It would be naive of any politician, pressure group, or administrator to think that any one country can implement this health strategy on its own. Many of the most deep-seated problems and new diseases can be tackled only at an international level through cooperation between individual countries and institutions throughout the European Region. The EEC has found that real cooperation works best through flexibility and a varying response from individual countries working in harness, held together by compelling issues rather than rules. This is how the Strategy will be implemented in the WHO European Region.

Because the Strategy can attract people right across the political spectrum, it offers an exciting prospect of new efforts in international cooperation. Heads of governments together could give a lead, which might take various forms, starting perhaps with a commitment to the aims drawn up at the Alma-Ata Conference for a global effort on primary health care. Alternatively, it may be more suitable at this stage to work at the European level and later link up with the rest of the world.

The areas that need international action include smoking, alcohol and infant foods (particularly in relation to promotion and distribution), drug trafficking, control of cross-frontier infections, food quality, and the side effects of tourism and aviation. There is specific work to be done on these and considerable benefits can accrue by cooperation in research, information, monitoring, and legislation.

One example of how countries throughout Europe, whatever their political differences, can cooperate is in the control by code and legislation of sulfur pollution from coal-burning power plants. Countries pollute the air of other countries indiscriminately. Some countries export vast amounts of sulfur dioxide that poison the lakes and rivers of other states, killing fish and exacerbating respiratory diseases through acid rain. The Organisation for Economic Co-operation and Development has shown, for example, that the United Kingdom in 1974 emitted 18 000 tons of sulfur deposits but received only about 10 000 tons, in effect dumping its wastes in other countries. Norway, by contrast, emitted about 400 tons but the rest of the Region dumped another 2500 tons on her (1). One of the problems about oilspills in the European Region is that no one affected can take action against the responsible ship at sea, and the government of registration to whom the spill may be reported may not be interested. Here again, international action is required.

Our planet is a closed system. All human activity involves waste but we have only one piece of land — the planet Earth. In the end, the waste catches up with us. We must therefore include the cost of waste in our calculations for the future, whether budgetary or legal, and we must take action to deal with it within the only framework possible — that of international collaboration. One way of starting this collaboration is through WHO's technical networks, which are described in the section on WHO's coordinating role (p. 150).

Finally, though this is a strategy for the WHO European Region, it has global implications for the movement for attaining health for all by the year 2000. There need be no dispute about the targets that must be adopted to reduce preventable conditions caused by alcohol, tobacco, road accidents, or failure to immunize. Unemployment is also a European and global problem and, if tackled with the health element in mind, can be taken as an issue into every international forum. The elderly, the blind, all the target groups of society deserve a hearing and subsequent action in the forums that are already available — the European Parliament, the Council of Europe, the Nordic Council, the Council for Mutual Economic Assistance.

TARGETS AND TIMETABLES

Targets there must be, and as the Strategy is brought together in its different national forms the stage should be set for a common political commitment of nations to work together, perhaps by the acceptance of a joint declaration by heads of government. It is only in this way that progress can really be monitored and timetables kept. Talk of an interdependent world has no meaning unless leaders are ready to take specific steps to give interdependence reality and carry their people along with them.

LEGISLATION BY PUBLIC DEMAND

The Strategy for Attaining Health for All by the Year 2000 will require legislation and new approaches. To prevent food poisoning most countries already have much legislation, but too little public education and enforcement. Food legislation, however, will illustrate the range of action needed. Pollution may need codes of practice reinforced by laws inflicting severe fines on offenders. For both, and for cigarettes, alcohol, infant foods, tourism, air travel, the control of chemicals, and the tracking down of disease, cooperation among countries on enforceable international regulations is needed.

Laws to help change

Lifestyles are usually a reflection not only of the individual's activities but also of the social structures and the pressures they impose. It is not enough to have voluntary codes for the alcohol or tobacco industry; extensive legislation is needed, as confirmed by experience in Finland. As early as 1961 the Finnish Parliament had called for strong measures against smoking but to little effect — voluntary restrictions on advertising and uncoordinated health education activities showed few results. Finally, in 1976, an Act to restrict tobacco smoking was passed. This rules that 0.5% of tobacco tax revenue must be set aside for developing a health-oriented tobacco policy. Advertising and sales promotion of tobacco were prohibited in 1978. The Government fixes limits on the tar, nicotine and carbon monoxide content of tobacco. A health warning is printed on all retail packages and the sale of tobacco to persons under 16 is forbidden. Smoking itself is also prohibited in all public places and on public transport except in separate areas. The massive publicity that surrounded the Government's policy and the Tobacco Act confirmed the Norwegian experience that the public debate itself contributed to change (2).

Obsolete laws governing the rights and duties of various groups in the existing medical profession may also be a hindrance to introducing new systems of primary medical care based on a participating community. Enabling legislation will be needed to cope with this and related areas such as budget control, and social security systems must be changed to emphasize prevention rather than payment for cure.

Because it would probably be counterproductive to impose health legislation (as opposed to controls on the cigarette industry) it must be clear exactly what legislation should do in the area of public opinion and lifestyles. Social pressure may lead people to realize that the combination of drinking and driving is dangerous, so that people begin to think before they do it. If they cause an accident because they do not they must pay the penalty imposed by law.

The social change in lifestyles will need to be accompanied in certain areas, however, by changes which can be achieved only by specific legislation. Good examples are smoking or drinking. As long as people are constantly exposed to persuasive sales promotion for alcohol and cigarettes, change is difficult. Governments, which receive vast revenues from or actually own alcohol or tobacco manufactories, must not have one law for themselves and one for private industry. A WHO expert committee has drawn up a list of proposed laws in this regard (3).

Laws that work

Public participation can be a great help in making sure that laws are passed and are effective. This is true for legislation concerning the movement and preparation of food. There is a mass of legislation in this area, but it has not been properly applied. There are too few food inspectors and they are often unnecessarily severe. Inspectors need to tell people in the food-handling business how to avoid food contamination (for most contamination is unwitting), and so promote good hygiene actively. They must also reach the home and school, so that people learn how to handle convenience foods.They can offer advice on new processes such as microwave cooking, and they can help ensure that any legislation required is up to date. Traders who deal in inferior foodstuffs have to be caught and punished. However, most people need advice and this can best be set down through a framework of food safety laws that are easy to understand and apply.

This kind of framework is needed for international cooperation on food legislation. It would be foolish to draft detailed model laws internationally and then try to apply them in each country. Each nation has its different approach to the preparation of food, the result of hundreds of years of experience and usually suited to its climate and conditions.

In relation to primary care, Finland has set the pace with its Primary Health Act of 1972. This made possible a complete reorganization of primary care based on health centres, and also introduced a new type of formal health planning. The health centre is the basic primary care unit, providing general practitioner, occupational health, maternal and child health, school health, child dental care and physiotherapy services for 10 000 or more people. The system now covers the whole country, with a total of 218 health centres. Cooperation among the primary care services, the specialist outpatient services and the hospitals ought to be very close, since they are all run by the same local authorities. Within the resources and guidance of an overall national plan, health plans are produced by the local authorities. Data collected and processed locally are included in the plans sent to the central authorities, who process regional and national data for the use of the local and district authorities. It is just this sort of legislative framework, which allows for planning from the bottom up and local participation and control, that will best ensure health for all.

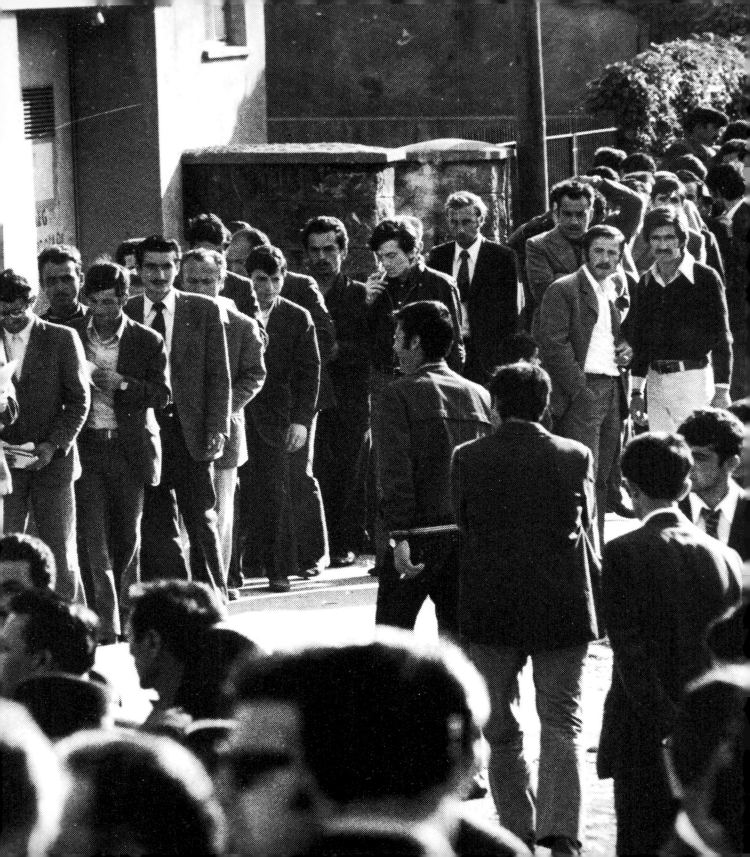

12.

The health cost of unemployment

The recession that is sweeping across Europe is already raising the spectre of incipient poverty. There is understandable fear that mass unemployment, exaggerated by the effects of new unplanned and un-controllable technology, will re-emerge. At the end of 1980 there were already some 10 million known unemployed in the EEC alone, and perhaps a third more who have kept out of, or should one say, not yet fallen into, the statistical maw? This figure would be much higher if account were also taken of "disguised unemployment", i.e., two or three workers doing the job that one worker could do. The detrimental effect of unemployment or "underemployment" on health has not been properly measured. A pilot study has, however, revealed a higher incidence of depression, asthma, headache, and backache among people who cannot get work (1).

Much of the success of the Strategy depends upon people choosing healthier lifestyles, but the choice of a new lifestyle is an empty one if it is severely limited by unemployment and poverty.

Poverty is relative and taints all those it touches. The comfortable family, whose breadwinner loses work, is forced to change its lifestyle and the choices that follow, in attempts to overcome stress, may often be unwise. The pressure to keep up appearances may be as damaging to some as near destitution would be to others. Many formerly well-off mothers may go hungry themselves to see their children well fed. Old people may scrimp on food, even to the extent of suffering from vitamin deficiencies, in order to buy decent clothes to wear before the neighbours. How much does unemployment cause mental and physical illness? How much does it lead to disruptive behaviour by young people who feel they have been betrayed or cheated of the chance to earn a good living? In some parts of the Region the television set, the refrigerator, and the washing machine may be luxuries; in others, their loss, or the pressure to keep up payments for them during unemployment, are pressures to be added to a home where there is fear that all the future can bring is more problems and no solutions (1). Whatever form it takes, every country, individually and in cooperation with its neighbours, must take action to counter unemployment. The whole community, from local to international level, is deeply involved in such action.

UNEMPLOYMENT KILLS

The latest evidence shows that the worse off you are, the more you are ill and the quicker you die (2). It used to be the great gap between the small number of the rich and the mass of the poor that made this so obvious. Now studies of statistics in the United States, and in England

and Wales between 1936 and 1976 (*3*), have shown that suicide and murder rates increased within a year of the increase in unemployment, while deaths from heart diseases began to increase 2–3 years after and the effect persisted for 10–15 years.

In modern Europe poverty is still part of the fabric of society, from the slums of Liverpool to the shanty towns of Naples. The redistribution of wealth through increased earning power over the last 30 years, however, has softened the impact of the great divide. Until recently, it was hard to see exactly where comfort and security ended and uncertainties and instability at home and work began to lead to poverty. There are clear and unjustifiable gaps between the rich and poor areas of the European Region, between the wealthy North and the poorer South. However, that comforting phrase "welfare state", combined with some ultimate certainty of government intervention in times of personal or community disaster, has slung a safety net beneath the public and the politicians and lulled them into a false sense of security.

That great divide is re-emerging in a more insidious form and brings with it illness of every kind, from depression to suicide (*4,5*), at once palliated and aggravated by alcoholism, wife and child battering, and bitterness. It spawns violence among the young, breaks up the home, precipitates divorce; it leads to poor diet, unhealthy children, and increased deaths among the newborn; people live in poor, perhaps damp, unheated accommodation, harassed by creditors, government bureaucrats and traders alike. There is a fundamental issue which has to be decided before we go further.

Unemployment hits the headlines — and hits at health. The newspaper cuttings over the page are from the 1980s. The following quotation ". . . the serious and extensive disturbances in social and economic life which are now occurring give rise to apprehension as to the consequences to health . . ." is taken from the Bulletin of the Health Organisation of the League of Nations, in 1932. (6)

Augustine's Abbey: The public are not welcome.

Graduates join dole queues

by AURIOL STEVENS
Education Correspondent

ONE IN FIVE new graduates could be out of a job this year, according to the Department of *Employment Gazette*.

The rising tide of economic depression now seems to have reached the graduate cohort, though graduates still remain the most favoured new entrants to the labour market, Neil Scott, director of the careers advisory service at Nottingham University says.

After many years of high graduate employment, it looks as if the troubles that have long afflicted American, Italian and Indian graduates are heading Britain's way.

There will be a 6 per cent rise in the number of graduates this year, but no increase is expected in the number of jobs available. About 15 per cent of last year's graduates are still jobless.

Forecasts last year over-estimated the likely number of jobs for new graduates by 20 per cent. Employers stopped recruiting as the recession deepened. Forecasts for this year are more tentative.

Electronics, the oil industry, banking, insurance and chartered accountancy are among the most promising areas. Vacancies in engineering, metals, retailing, the Civil Service—apart from the Armed Forces, the police and some parts of the scientific civil service—are all down.

Graduates with science degrees are better placed than those with arts or sociology degrees,

Historic monuments are closed by freeze on jobs

by PETER DEELEY

TWENTY - ONE historic monuments in the care of the Department of the Environment have been closed to the public because of a freeze on staff recruitment.

They include major tourist attractions such as St Augustine's Abbey in Canterbury, English church, near Hastings...

...scholars and local authorities for whom the sites bring both fame and trade. Historians and researchers fear that unless the sites are protected, vandalism and the depredations of the weather will cause irrevocable damage.

An estimated 11 million people visit Britain's monuments each year, paying £4.7 million in entrance fees where there is a charge.

The Inspectorate of Ancient Monuments employs 145 custodians and 73 part-time care-takers on the staff of the Environ-ment...

...MP for Holborn and St Pancras. Who has raised the question of the erosion of Britain's heritage with Mr Michael Heseltine, the Environment Secretary, said: 'These closures are both short-sighted and damaging. Ruins quickly become irreparable if they are not watched over.

In Norfolk at least two monuments are now shut, the eleventh century Castle Acre, built for the son-in-law of William the Conqueror, Castle Acre was handed to the Government earlier this century on the understanding that it should be kept open for the public benefit.

Solicitors for the former...have written to Mr Richard...asking for...

Junior do face dole

CHRISTINE DOYLE

SIVE unemployment junior doctors, anied by even waiting lists and standards of treatinevitable unless ment makes it juniors to of their pro-arliamentary be told this

...among the hospital militancy, sultan chair-medical Staff of the...

...to run a Parliament based on ining rather will be to oper number to allow for ultants. The consultants ent and not patients' li Dr Rees. more than stem, he be about junior doc

ears ago an aver-
[abou]t 40 people per
[pati]ents killed them-
under the care of
[hospi]tals. By the 1970s
[a]verage had risen
[ov]er 100,000.

Sainsbury, re-
[directo]r of the Medical
[cou]ncil psychiatric
[...]gwell Hospital,
said : 'These
[m]ost certainly
the problem.
[...] patients were
[s]trictly super-
that the cur-
[li]beral hostel
[les]s supervision
[r]eason for the

[...]ewson-Smith,
[psychi]atrist at the
[...] in Hamp-
the supervi-

---

sion of patients in the new
general hospital units which
have replaced the big mental
hospital was more difficult.

A [...]chia[...]
the [...]
agreed [...]
distu[...]
Rich[...]
comm[...]
min[...]
poir[...]
diff[...]
a n[...]

By David Felton
Labour Reporter

Mr James Prior, Secretary of State for Employment, issued a warning last night that there would be another "very big" rise in unemployment this month and the trend of the "appalling" jobless figures was likely to continue.

[cou]pled the warning with [...] Govern-

tinue into the year, although we do expect it to ease off as time goes on". But these [...] figures are, sadly, the inevitable consequence of many years of decline, of a failure of past attempts to reverse that decline.

As an indication of the Government's concern at levels of unemployment, Mr Prior pointed in particular to the [...]portunities programme; [...] 440,000

Doling out disease

David Ennals, former social services secretary, writes on the association between ill health and unemployment. He anticipates serious problems in the coming years, as unemployment rises

Lord Nelson's comment that "harbour rots good ships and good men" is as true today as when he said it. It is generally accepted that long term unemployment, particularly among family men, contributes towards mental ill-health, male suicide, family breakdowns and child abuse.

However, uncertain[...] our knowledge about the effects of unemployment on health. For example, to what extent is the effect of unemployment exacerbated by poverty. Many if not most unemployed people lack savings. Earnings related benefits – soon to cease – only last six months and only a few are eligible for them. A family with two children now receives £38 a week in unemployment benefits plus £10.50 in child benefits and housing help. Supplementary benefit is only slightly high-er. The Child Poverty Action Group and the Family Service Units recently showed that without incurring debts, families on sup-plementary benefits could not afford sufficient food, heating and clothing. Result: stress and, in some cases, ill health.

Thus it is difficult to divorce the effects of unemployment from the effects of very low income. Interestingly, the Black Report (1980) on inequalities in health – with its social class comparisons – hardly considered the effects of [un]employment. This was because the statistics [...] available showed that the jobless [acc]ounted for a relatively small proportion of [the] population.

[Fu]rthermore when the number of unem-[ployed] hovered around the million mark, [...] people were able to change one job for [...] fairly quickly. Now that one in seven [of the] male labour force is out of work, [...]gistered unemployed worker [... on] average, to be jobl[...]

an ever increasing number may never work again.

How high will unemployment go and how long will it take to drop? Estimates vary, but none of the forecasters, on the basis of current Government policy, predict a fall in the next two or three years.

What about the effect of job loss? A 1980 Gallup poll reported that the number of peo-ple fearing for their jobs had risen from 27 per cent in June to 38 per cent in September. These were justifiable fears: since then unem-ployment is up by a million. Many people are similarly preoccupied today, parti-cularly schoolchildren who must wonder if they will ever work at all.

I know of no research into the fears of unemployment. In fact, in a study of "stress" I published in 1973, I made only passing refer-ence to the effect of fears of job loss on employment. One could conclude that the cur-rent decrease in sickness absence indicates the benefit of economic uncertainty. My own view is that the opposite is the case and that the fear of sickness induced absence from work is keeping people away from GPs and making them neglect their health.

In fact, I don't know if this is the case. Similarly, many other theories and conclusions from studies are inevitably tentative and open to challenge. Much depends upon interpreta-tion of data. For example, Dr [...] Vaughan has been challenged [...] sentation to Parliament [...] study, Unemploy[...] have [...]

USA and the UK. Professor Brenner strongly defended his thesis linking the unem-ployment rate to heart disease, sclerosis of the liver and even suicide.

Scepticism also marks another DHSS report (Unemployment Gazette, volume 98) about the changing health of 2,300 men sacked in 1978. This does not dispute the association between unemployment and ill health but it suggests that unhealthy people are more likely than others to lose their jobs and less likely to find new ones; and that those who join the ranks of the unemployed are more likely to [...] and badly housed.

I believe the true [...] emerge from [...] from [...]

---

s
[...]
ue

[in]deci[...]
Pati[...]
tim[...]
to l[...]
sf[...]
al[...]

THE CHEATING BRIBE

Are we paying people to be idle because they cannot get work, and therefore encouraging them to sit around because they can be "better off" on the dole, or is the richer, stronger, and now larger, part of society — the part that has the skills and is the fittest to survive — really exploiting the 10, 15 or 20 per cent of society who carry the *real* burden of economic recession? Closer examination would seem to indicate that this is exactly what we are doing.

Most of society and particularly, of course, politicians must take the responsibility for this. They are actually swinging a very satisfactory deal for themselves. In return for a survival payment, the unemployed are being compelled to shoulder the burden of everyone else's insecurity.

They are also being asked to see their children develop into the next generation of unemployed: literally whole classes on the dole, who will have missed out on the first job market when leaving school and who will never catch up with their peers. Schools are now giving final-year students courses on how to cope if they cannot find a job. Unemployed parents, whose children are still at school, see them losing educational opportunities because of the pressures on the home. Children still in the womb will be born less healthy, and will be affected by their parents' heavier drinking.

It is the weaker group which has to face continual economic instability and insecurity, reaching crisis levels during recessions. It is in recession that women's jobs first go to the wall. The people in those industries whose goods are not essential are the first to lose their jobs and the last to get them back.

GUARANTEED UNEMPLOYMENT?

The next twist is that when recession abates it is more than likely that the jobs of the unskilled will no longer exist. This is normal in any modern industrial society, but the problem is going to be much worse in the future because of the microchip revolution, unless it is planned for. That seems unlikely, judging by the way we are failing to find radical solutions to the present unemployment.

We are also building up another kind of unemployment based on disability. Consumer demands for cheaper, more varied products, and the factory owners' response to that, catch us in a trap. Increasing pressure is put on workers to increase productivity, but we are not monitoring what this is doing to society as a whole. There is greater and greater stress on the individual in the name of efficiency, and now we hear of early retirement through disability or migraines or bad hearts. How often has this been because we have actually manufactured ill health at the conveyor belt? How often does someone retire after a nervous breakdown because he can no longer cope with the lonely responsibility of manning a computer panel which controls a whole power plant or steel works?

We have made it possible for one person to do the work of 20 or 30 or even hundreds — but how much have we increased stress on that one man? These people may be living on their early retirement and disablement pension (if one is available), but that is simply another kind of unemployment benefit with all the accompanying ills.

Unemployment, therefore, spreads out from the breadwinner to the whole community, leading to major social problems for which there are no simple cosmetic answers. Society must intervene or it will do itself severe long-term damage. What is more, it must intervene in a way that does not simply export the problem of unemployment to poorer regions within Europe or to the developing world. The recession and its effects cannot be seen as isolated problems affecting only part of the globe. The public and the politicians must come up with major answers and be ready to take action.

There may be some short-term answers which could help lessen the devastating long-term effects on individuals and communities. There has been much talk about job sharing. There is a tendency to self-protection here; the man with the job feels threatened. However, not only is he paying someone else to carry the burden of unemployment — he is paying it out of his taxes anyway. There would seem to be some way for government, the taxman and the public to work out a formula so that the tax payment could keep somone in work instead.

The major decisions and shifts in approach that need to be taken are going to demand relevant information, and we do not have enough. Research into the whole background of unemployment and its effects would certainly show those in doubt what it is not too hard to realize already: unemployment does not pay anybody anything, least of all the politician who thinks he is saving "public money" by not supporting an industry with subsidies and by paying dole instead. Politicians are often accused of not thinking in the long term. The next generation of young voters will bring with them bitterness against those leaders who have failed to meet the challenge and have asked the young to carry the cross for everyone else. There is no guarantee for those politicians that the young will accept this for ever.

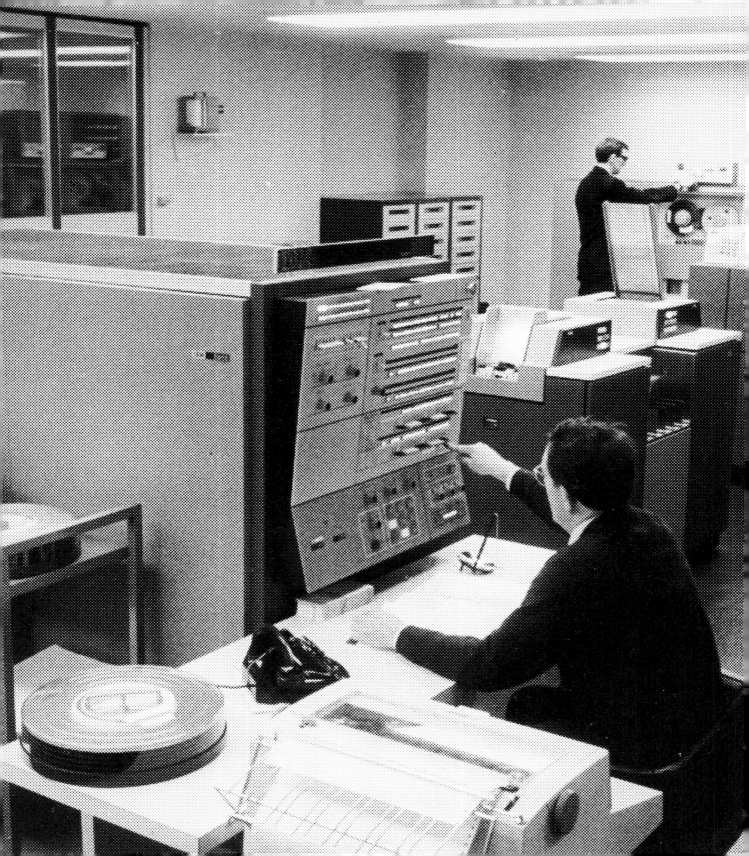

13.

Information, research and monitoring

Information, research, and monitoring are crucial factors at the local, national, and international level and are needed to cover the three areas of the Strategy: health as a way of life, the battle to prevent ill health, and a community care system that is appropriate, accessible, and adequate.

SPREADING THE WORD

Because the involvement of the community is a key ingredient, people should have access to information. The media can play an important role, but new ways of using traditional social networks to spread information are needed. These networks may be schools, but they may also be care groups such as Alcoholics Anonymous, social groups, youth clubs, sporting associations, or pressure groups. The medium of advertising must also be harnessed in the promotion of health as a way of life. Every aspect of public life needs to take health into account, so civil servants are a target group requiring easy access to information that is easy to apply.

New information will become available to us only if society, through governments, is prepared to back the necessary research, whether in universities or among particular groups involved in health care. Laboratory testing conditions are good for some things, but some knowledge will be found only in people's everyday lives. Hence their involvement is essential. For example, the people who best know the health of children are their mothers, but too often mother and doctor fail to capitalize on this. We have not succeeded in working out why smoking, alcoholism, and drug addiction are so difficult to treat. Our understanding of the effects of unemployment and its personal and full financial cost is incomplete. So that we can anticipate them and provide for them, we need to know more about the diseases of old age. The long-term effects of pollution of every kind will certainly catch us unawares unless we begin to try to understand the bewildering number of factors that influence us and life around us.

TECHNOLOGY FOR ALL

Technological research has brought great benefits but it can bring even more if it is coordinated, made cost-effective, and spread widely in an imaginative way. Thus, the electronic computer, which has been expensive to develop, is now fast becoming a highly effective and cheap adjunct to everyday life, invaluable for a multitude of different jobs. Technological research must, however, be accompanied by early warning systems on the look-out for defects that will be costly later.

There is a particular role for industry itself in the development of medical equipment. The community, including the health professions, must use its new knowledge to tell industry what it wants to see developed and governments must ensure that the basic rules of the Strategy are observed in this context. A new range of sophisticated battery- or mains-powered electronic equipment could be developed for primary health care, either for professionals in health centres or for home use. We should have no fear of health technology whether as users or medical professionals. The development of techniques that allow us to investigate the body without "invading" it and so causing wounds, as a needle does for example, has removed one of the biggest obstacles to nonprofessionals doing investigations. We already have the use, although generally only in hospitals, of endoscopy, ultrasound, and computer-assisted tomography (CAT) — the body scanner. The miniaturization and simplification of much equipment would also expand the diagnostic role of health professionals such as nurses, who so far have been regarded mainly as helpers to doctors, not people who can take over many of the routine roles of the physician. There is no question of replacing the doctor, but his knowledge can be better employed as a catalyst, or he can perhaps play the role of team leader.

NORTH ⇋ SOUTH

The move towards primary health care is worldwide, but the resources for technological development are still found mainly in the industrialized countries. These should recognize their responsibility for sharing new knowledge with other regions of the world and should transfer technology. However, Europe can also benefit from many of the ideas that have emerged through necessity in developing countries. For example, their populations have been recycling resources for years and have learnt how to make the best of the often meagre resources that were available. Developing countries can learn from the mistakes of developed countries. If developing countries can use new, cheap, sophisticated technology and bypass the early stages, they will have the chance to tackle some of the problems that Europe left them at the end of the colonial era. One opportunity would be to employ satellites for spreading the range of television. For a developing country it would be inestimably cheaper to put up or share a satellite for transmission, than to build ground relay stations across the country. The satellite television experiment in India showed this. Through battery-powered sets and chicken-mesh aerials to pick up the satellite signal, India provided television to thousands of villages that often had no electricity. Battery-powered apparatus in the hands of a village health worker for blood analysis to detect malaria parasites would make a dramatic difference to millions of people.

At the moment there are huge numbers of unexamined blood-slides in many countries because they do not have the laboratories or the manpower to deal with them. Europe is making available its training facilities for such work but can do much more. In the field of pharmaceutical and vaccine production, various WHO-coordinated reference and quality control schemes involving collaboration among laboratories on a worldwide basis could be extended (*1,2*).

FEEDBACK FOR PROGRESS

Research results need evaluation, a task that will differ from country to country. An essential for all countries, however, is exchange of information. A basic framework for a health policy for the whole of Europe will never exist unless the information that becomes available is put to use by all countries. Computer technology gives us a new chance to cope with the volume of information that will develop. The advent of simple computers means that local health centres will be able to provide vital detailed information (which can be kept confidential) about their patients' health without becoming bogged down in paperwork. The aim is to make the information widely available to every sector of society and use it to make sensible decisions. At present small groups of specialists ponder over data and proposals and report to even smaller groups of people who may then take decisions for hundreds of thousands of people.

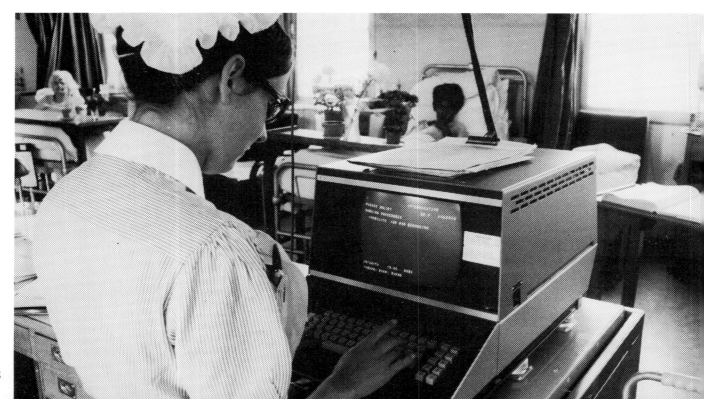

THE COORDINATING ROLE OF WHO

International organizations often come in for criticism, WHO and its Regional Offices being no exception. WHO has, however, assumed a new role in recent years, combining expertise and common sense to make a real contribution to the daily lives of millions. It is this new role that has become a hallmark and given WHO the courage to venture into areas where others, including governments, have never dared set foot. Thus, it has brought together pressure groups on the one hand and manufacturers of baby foods on the other. Baby-food manufacturers are among the most powerful multinational corporations in the world, with resources far beyond those of many of the world's nations. Yet because of its reputation for expertise and straightforwardness WHO has been able to persuade pressure groups and food companies to agree on a code of practice in the promotion of these products.

The WHO Regional Office for Europe has been responsible for pulling together the many strands of government, medical, and expert opinion leading to the realization that a whole new health strategy is needed for the Region. It will, in the same way, help in the formulation of the plans and programmes needed to give effect to that strategy. Thus, a series of legislative measures will be needed in the Member States, each with its own different emphasis. The Regional Office has already started to build a comparative framework for the health legislation of different countries, which will enable Member States to turn to it to find out what has been done by other countries and save much time (1).

The Regional Office is already the central reference point for the Strategy, and as information grows it can ensure that it is collected in the most useful form and properly analysed, and that it reaches those who need to use it to make decisions. It has already begun mapping out a series of programmes and targets for countries to aim at if they are to tackle the root causes of our new diseases. Combined political action will need to be taken on the basis of those programmes at the highest level and throughout the entire Region.

WHO is concerned to see that not only governments and the professions but also pressure groups and the public are informed. These groups should feel able to turn to WHO for objective technical support in the same way as the medical profession has been able to turn to it in the past. This is not a change of role but a natural progression as the realization grows that community care means more than just curative medicine. Groups seeking changes in smoking habits and legislation can draw on the material WHO has already brought together in publications embodying the best expert opinion available in the field.

Highly effective electronic computers can now be made so small, simple and cheap, that they can transform a wide variety of everyday tasks. On the ward, nurse has clear up-to-date information on all her patients at her fingertips.

WHO can also act as an impartial source of assessment for the development of new technologies. It does not necessarily have the resources itself to make assessments but it has developed a network of independent experts that can. In the same way it can offer a reference point for the standardization of equipment so that different parts of the Region can buy similar easily maintained and serviced equipment. It can also ensure that outdated technology from one area is not peddled to another.

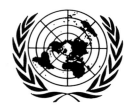

Within the global role of WHO's Strategy for Attaining Health for All by the Year 2000 the European Region can ensure that developing countries do not commit the mistakes many European countries have committed. One of the best offerings to the developing world is probably a clear explanation of such mistakes and how they can be avoided. As most of the resources for the development of medicine — equipment, men and money — are still located in the European Region, that imposes a grave responsibility. Another is to make sure that research also benefits the developing world. Too many health services in Europe have been content to man their operations with the brains of doctors and nurses who were most needed in developing countries themselves. Whatever the attractions, money or better research facilities, Europe must begin to recognize that imbalance for what it is — the rich gaining at the expense of the poor — and begin to assess how it should change.

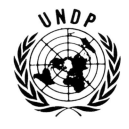

Finally, the WHO Regional Office for Europe cannot simply act as a nerve centre for new training courses, or improved models of primary health care. It would be a gross dereliction of its duty if it did not also act as a conscience for the Region. There will be times when it must point the finger at the public, at government or at industry as the case may be. If a watchdog group comes to it for advice, perhaps in the support of a parliamentary investigation, the WHO Regional Office for Europe is there to offer that advice, sure in the professional knowledge that it is not taking sides but simply helping search for the truth.

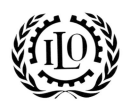

Collaborative mechanisms
Some of the specific areas mentioned in the Strategy document about WHO's co-ordinating role are as follows.

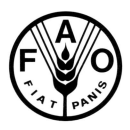

A Regional Health Development Advisory Council has been set up, including representatives of health and other sectors. This group has been heavily involved in advising the Regional Director on the formulation of the Strategy for Attaining Health for All by the Year 2000. It will help follow up the implementation of the Strategy and provide the Regional Committee (composed of representatives of the 33 Member States) with the relevant information for evaluation, coordination and corrective action.

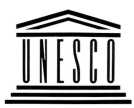

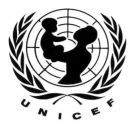

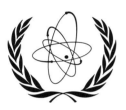

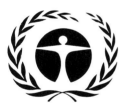

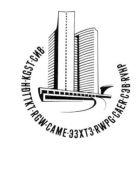

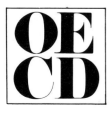

The Organization has a clearly defined role in the joint relief and rehabilitation efforts undertaken by the United Nations system and the League of Red Cross Societies with regard to disasters and natural catastrophes. For such eventualities the Regional Office has direct relations with nongovernmental organizations interested in disaster relief, will maintain a roster of experts available at short notice, and will develop standards for prompt intervention. Contingency planning is already under way at the regional level for emergencies involving the release of toxic chemicals into the environment.

Contacts and joint meetings with the 30 or more nongovernmental organizations in the Region with which WHO collaborates at present, and particularly with associations for medical education, associations of schools of public health, and professional associations, may be used to facilitate an understanding and the implementation of the Strategy.

The recognition, by the United Nations General Assembly, of health as an integral part of development will be reflected in the future collaborative activities at country level with other United Nations agencies and at regional level with the United Nations Economic Commission for Europe (ECE). Collaboration with these other bodies is already close: the United Nations Development Programme (UNDP) and other agencies are invited to all programming meetings and Regional Office officials participate in UNDP country programme reviews. Major benefits in health and social sectors could be expected from a joint planning mechanism, to be established in collaboration with ECE.

Intercountry collaboration
Intercountry collaboration in the European Region is supported by several subregional intergovernmental organizations. The Regional Office will continue to ensure collaboration in the health field by inviting representatives of these organizations to programming meetings, and by participating in joint activities. Technical cooperation among countries will be developed by making more extensive use of available information, exchanging teachers and students, coordinating the production and testing of equipment and drugs, and exchanging expertise, especially through intercountry collaborating centres for research programmes related to the Regional Strategy.

Interregional collaboration
The European Region already plays an important role in interregional exchanges, and particularly in North ⇌ South cooperation, either on a bilateral or multilateral basis. The European countries and intergovernmental organizations should be involved in all machinery set up in other regions and at global level for the mobilization of resources for poorer countries. For many aspects of health development, the experiences of Europe, positive and negative, are often the lessons to help speed up development processes in other parts of the world. These need to be properly analysed, evaluated and published. The Regional Office, in liaison with headquarters, should play a coordinating role, making available information on needs and resources, supporting the use of research and training in European institutions, and encouraging interregional meetings and the participation of other regions in meetings organized in Europe.

Photo credits   Front cover: WHO. Frontispiece: Tom Luke.   **Chapter 1** facing page 1: Kaj Lund Hansen. page 7: WHO/Jean Mohr. page 11: UNESCO/Dominique Roger. page 17: WHO/Agerpress Photo.   **Chapter 2**   page 18: Menne/Bavaria. page 25 top: Edo König/Bavaria. page 25 bottom: Oscar Poss/Bavaria. page 29: Jan Unger. page 35: WHO/E. Mandelmann.   **Chapter 3**   page 38: Piotr. page 41: WHO. page 43: Klaus Meier-Ude/Bavaria. page 45: Gunvor Jørgsholm. page 47: Erik Kragh.   **Chapter 4**   page 50: Per Brogaard. page 53: Kaj Lund Hansen. page 55: WHO/P. Almasy. page 57: Helle Nielsen. page 59: Christian Lotzbeck. page 61: United Nations/Muldoon jr.   **Chapter 5**   page 64: Tom Luke. page 68: Peeters Monique – Duffel. page 71: WHO/Jean Mohr. page 73: WHO/E. Mandelmann.   **Chapter 6**   page 74: Steen Mansson. page 79: WHO/Eric Schwab. page 81: Kaj Lund Hansen. page 82: Manfred Below/Bavaria. page 83: Bjarne Geiges/Bavaria.   **Chapter 7**   page 84: FAO/Camillo Boscardi. page 87: Pierre Berger/Bavaria. page 89: Distilled Spirits Council of the United States, Inc. (DISCUS). page 93: Kræftens Bekæmpelse.   **Chapter 8**   page 94: Bo Jarner. page 98 left: Torsten Graae. page 98 right: WHO/UNICEF/A. Duran. page 101: WHO/Jean Mohr. page 104: Hans Schmied/Bavaria. page 107: Klaus Meier-Ude/Bavaria. page 111: WHO/Eric Schwab.   **Chapter 9**   page 112: Bo Jarner. page 116: WHO/E. Mandelmann. page 119: ILO/J. Maillard.   **Chapter 10**   page 120: Piotr. page 125: United Nations/J. Slaughter.   **Chapter 11**   page 126: Tom Luke. page 129: Ebbe Andersen.   **Chapter 12**   page 136: ILO.   **Chapter 13**   page 145: WHO/Tibor Farkas. page 149: WHO/P. Larsen.

References

Origins of the impending crisis

1. *Health care in the Netherlands. Financial analysis 1973–1983.* Leidschendam, Ministry of Health and Environmental Protection, 1979.
2. *The problem of medical technology.* Copenhagen, WHO Regional Office for Europe, 1980 (unpublished document R4/48/2(30)).
3. *Health services in Europe,* 3rd ed. Copenhagen, WHO Regional Office for Europe, 1981.
4. **Kaprio, L.A.** *Primary health care in Europe.* Copenhagen, WHO Regional Office for Europe, 1979 (EURO Reports and Studies, No. 14).
5. **Field, F,** *Inequality in Britain.* Glasgow, Fontana Paperbacks, 1981.
6. **Lynge, E.** *Socio-economic differences in mortality in Europe.* Strasbourg, Council of Europe, 1980 (document ED-MM 3 (80) prov).
7. *Annual epidemiological and vital statistics. Part I. Vital statistics and causes of death,* 1955–1961. Geneva, World Health Organization.
8. *World health statistics annual. Vol. I. Vital statistics and causes of death,* 1962–1978. Geneva, World Health Organization.
9. *Inequalities in health.* London, Department of Health and Social Security, 1980.
10. **Brown, G.W. & Harris, T.** *Social origins of depression: a study of psychiatric disorder in women.* London, Tavistock, 1978.
11. **Ferguson, T.** Social support systems as self-care. *Medical self-care,* 7: 5 (1979).
12. **Abel-Smith, B.** Health care in a cold economic climate. *Lancet,* 1: 373–376 (1981).

The "New Diseases"

1. *Demographic yearbook.* New York, United Nations, 1977.
2. *Public health aspects of alcohol and drug dependence:* report on a WHO Conference. Copenhagen, WHO Regional Office for Europe, 1979 (EURO Reports and Studies, No. 8).
3. **Walsh, D.** *Alcohol-related medicosocial problems and their prevention.* Copenhagen, WHO Regional Office for Europe, 1982 (Public Health in Europe, No. 17).
4. **Willcox, R.R.** *The management of sexually transmitted diseases. A guide for the general practitioner.* Copenhagen, WHO Regional Office for Europe, 1979 (EURO Reports and Studies, No. 12).
5. *Life style related diseases – a major concern in Swedish health care planning.* Stockholm, Ministry of Health and Social Affairs, 1980 (unpublished document).
6. *Tobacco consumption in various countries,* 4th ed. London, Tobacco Research Council, 1975 (Research Paper, No. 6).
7. *Annual epidemiological and vital statistics. Part I. Vital statistics and*

causes of death, 1951. Geneva, World Health Organization.

8. *EURO programme profile: mental health.* Copenhagen, WHO Regional Office for Europe, 1979 (unpublished document).
9. *World health statistics annual. Vol. I. Vital statistics and causes of death,* 1965 and 1973. Geneva, World Health Organization.

Loss of caring in the community

1. **Kaprio, L.A.** *Primary health care in Europe.* Copenhagen, WHO Regional Office for Europe, 1979 (EURO Reports and Studies, No. 14).
2. **Mahler, H.** The meaning of "health for all by the year 2000". *World health forum,* **2**(1): 5–22 (1981).
3. **Vuori, H.** *Primary health care in industrialized countries.* Copenhagen, WHO Regional Office for Europe, 1980 (unpublished document).
4. *Health services in Europe,* 3rd ed. Copenhagen, WHO Regional Office for Europe, 1981, vol. 2, p. 114.

Self-care and consumer participation

1. **Mahler, H.** The meaning of "health for all by the year 2000". *World health forum,* **2**(1): 5–22 (1981).
2. **Parker, M.T., ed.** *Hospital-acquired infections: guidelines to laboratory methods.* Copenhagen, WHO Regional Office for Europe, 1978 (WHO Regional Publications, European Series, No. 4).
3. **Clemmesen, J.** *Statistical studies in malignant neoplasms.* Copenhagen, Munksgaard, 1977, vol. V.

New challenge for the health profession

1. **Mahler, H.** The meaning of "health for all by the year 2000". *World health forum,* **2**(1): 5–22 (1981).
2. **Härö, A.S.** *Country decision making for the achievement of the objective of primary health care.* Joint WHO/UNICEF JCHP Study: Case Study Finland, 1980 (unpublished document).
3. **Kaprio, L.A.** *Primary health care in Europe.* Copenhagen, WHO Regional Office for Europe, 1979 (EURO Reports and Studies, No. 14).

New health for all

1. *Psychogeriatric care in the community.* Copenhagen, WHO Regional Office for Europe, 1979 (Public Health in Europe, No. 10).
2. *World population trends and prospects by country, 1950–2000: summary report of the 1978 assessment.* New York, United Nations, 1979.

Health as a way of life

1. **Murray, L.** What are medical students learning about sexual medicine? Not enough, says Dr Harold I. Leif. *Sexual medicine today,* **5**(1): 6–13 (1981).
2. Practice on the fringe. *Update,* **23**(7): 921–924 (1981).
3. **Crawford, R.** Healthism and the medicalization of everyday life. *International journal of health services,* **10**(3): 365–388 (1980).
4. WHO Technical Report Series, No. 636, 1979 (*Controlling the smoking epidemic:* report of the WHO Expert Committee on Smoking Control).

The battle to prevent ill health

1. **Himmelberger, D.U. et al.** Cigarette smoking during pregnancy and the occurrence of spontaneous abortion and congenital abnormality. *American journal of epidemiology,* **108**(6): 470–479 (1978).
2. *Social indicators for the European Community 1960–1978.* Luxembourg, Statistical Office of the European Communities, 1980.
3. **Ziegler, P.N.** *Seat belt usage data collected from 19 countries.* Washington, DC, Department of Transportation, National Highway Traffic Safety Administration, 1979.
4. **Velimirovic, B.,** unpublished data.
5. *Food control laboratories.* Copenhagen, WHO Regional Office for Europe, 1978 (unpublished document ICP/FSP 003).
6. *Health aspects related to indoor air quality:* report on a WHO Working Group. Copenhagen, WHO Regional Office for Europe, 1979 (EURO Reports and Studies, No. 21).
7. **MRC Institute of Hearing Research.** Population study of hearing disorders in adults: preliminary communication. *Journal of the Royal Society of Medicine,* **74** (November 1981).
8. **Haggard, M. et al.** The high prevalence of hearing disorders and its implications for services in the UK. *British journal of audiology,* **15** (1981).

Community care means people

1. *Changing patterns in mental health care:* report on a WHO Working Group. Copenhagen, WHO Regional Office for Europe, 1980 (EURO Reports and Studies, No. 25).
2. **Elliott-Binns, C.P.** The first form of care. An analysis of lay medicine. *Journal of the Royal College of General Practitioners,* 23: 255–264 (1973).

Value for money

1. **Joarder, A.K. et al.** *The eradication of smallpox from Bangladesh.* New Delhi, WHO Regional Office for South-East Asia, 1980 (WHO Regional Publications, South-East Asia Series, No. 8).
2. **Basu, R.N. et al.** *The eradication of smallpox from India.* New Delhi, WHO Regional Office for South-East Asia, 1979 (WHO Regional Publications, South-East Asia Series, No. 5).
3. **Magee, J.** A windfall for development. *World health,* 5 (May 1980).

The role of politics

1. Steps towards controlling the "export" of air pollution. *OECD Observer,* 88: 6–8 (1977).
2. **Leppo, I.** Smoking control policy and legislation. *British medical journal,* 1: 343–347 (1978).
3. WHO Technical Report Series, No. 636, 1979 (*Controlling the smoking epidemic:* report of the WHO Expert Committee on Smoking Control).

The health cost of unemployment

1. **Fagin, L.** *Unemployment and health in families: case studies based on family interviews – a pilot study.* London, Department of Health and Social Security, 1981.
2. *Study on the influence of economic development on health:* report on a WHO Planning Meeting. Copenhagen, WHO Regional Office for Europe, 1981 (unpublished document ICP/RPD 804(1)).
3. **Brenner, M.H.** Mortality and the national economy. A review and the experience of England and Wales, 1936–1976. *Lancet,* 2(8142): 568–573 (1979).
4. **Thomas, K.B.** Waterlooville. *British medical journal,* 282: 1520 (1981).
5. **Colledge, M.** *Unemployment and health.* Tyne and Wear, United Kingdom, North Tyneside Community Health Council, 1981.

6. The economic depression and public health. *Quarterly bulletin of the Health Organisation,* **1**: 425–476 (1932).

Information, research and monitoring

1. **Akinyanju, P.A.** Quality control in developing countries. *Clinical chemistry news,* **1**: 131–133 (1981).
2. Report on the 1st African and Mediterranean Congress of Clinical Chemistry. *IFCC News,* **1**: 10–11 (1981).

The coordinating role of WHO

1. *Medium-term programme for health legislation.* Copenhagen, WHO Regional Office for Europe, 1980 (unpublished document).

LIST OF TABLES AND GRAPHS

LIST OF PHOTOS

WE HAVE BEEN CALLED UPON

We have been called upon
by statistics
in an average life
to open a very great number of
doors, tin cans
purses, wallets, checking accounts,
to close a very great number of
the same
except tin cans
to go by bus
car, bicycle, subway
to wear out shoes
butter bread
play ping-pong
yawn
feel glutted
chronically
statistically
glutted in the gut
the gutter between nausea
and vomit.

We have been called upon
to do away with accidental hunger
it's a fiction
the expectation
a fiction.
We are too busy opening
doors.

The thought of the times we shall
cross the street inside pedestrian crosswalks
outside pedestrian crosswalks
at stop lights
at intersections with live
policemen or
automatic policemen
stop signs
cause gastrointestinal
disturbances in the form of
gluttedness
the absence of hunger pangs
profuse acid secretion in
the stomach.

We have been called upon
through extensive knowledge of
human life
to die
from traffic accidents
of heart failure
arteriosclerosis

cancer
cancer
plus a series of other diseases

too special to die of
purely statistically.
But at a certain moment
in the series of door openings
it's proper to put
the clodhoppers
outside the specific cause
and swallow one's allotted death
which we have been glutted with throughout
our lives.

                                        Klaus Rifbjerg